Tomislav Birtić
I LOST 90 POUNDS FOR GOOD

TOMISLAV BIRTIĆ

I LOST

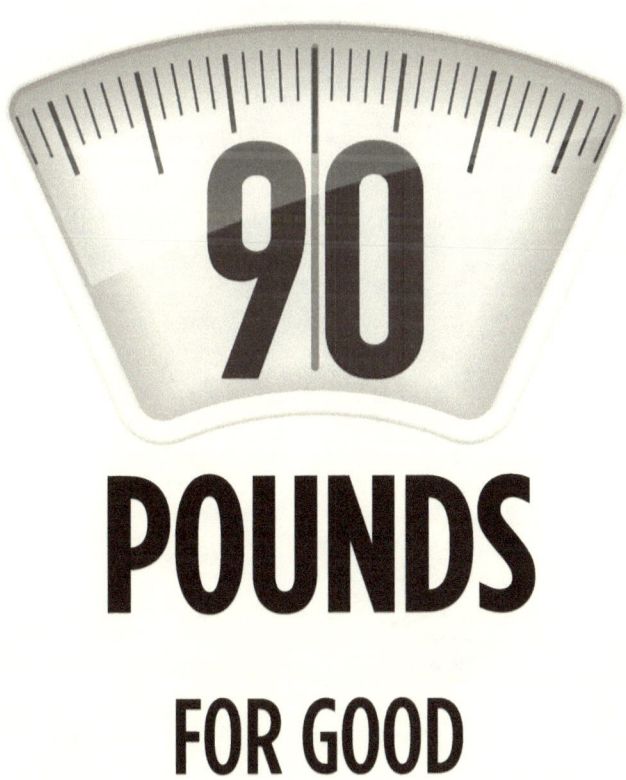

90

POUNDS

FOR GOOD

One of the greatest achievements of the human conscious is to be full, without eating

"Son, do you know anyone who walks everywhere who is fat?" – my father Nikola

UNDEAD, ONE STEP FROM DEATH

I could not feel the left side of my head, my left arm, nor my left leg. The little finger on my left hand seemed to be made of wood. I pinched it, but I couldn't feel anything, only the fingers of my right hand I was using to press it. I could not hear with my left ear. I put the headphones in my ear, I turned the sound up as loud as I could, but I couldn't hear anything at all. I was breathing in shallow breaths with enormous difficulty. I tried to take a deep breath. I couldn't do it. Something was squeezing me horribly in my chest. It didn't hurt (dully) as much as it scared me. Pure fear, fear of death, mixed with hope that perhaps it wasn't so bad, and searching for arguments acceptable to my mind, that everything would be fine.

I went out of the office, in front of the building. I leaned my palms on the metal fence. And waited for it to pass. And waited for it to pass. It didn't pass.

For weeks, months, it had been getting worse and worse. But, I thought, I comforted myself, it had been like this before. Stress. It had never been this bad, but it was nothing new to me. I only had to calm myself down. Everything would be alright. I suppose it would be alright. This onslaught of horrifying stress would pass too, and everything would be alright again.

I lit a cigarette. Blazing heat, more than 86 Fahrenheit (30 degrees), and a cigarette. For a few minutes

I walked up and down. It was no worse, nor any better. I went back to the office.

In three days I was going on holiday. I didn't tell my boss or my colleagues that I wasn't well. I intended to somehow get through those three days, to swim my heart out in the sea, as much as an out of shape man can.

Boris, my boss, my best friend, was sitting in front of me, my two colleagues, Renato and Zoran, to my right, and I spent the entire time looking straight to my left. In order to hear Boris, I had to turn to the left, turn my head away from him and them.

"Why won't you look at me while we are talking?" Boris asked.

"I can't hear with my left ear," I admitted.

"What! Are you OK?"

I admitted everything. Half my head, my left arm, my left leg, pressure in my chest...

"You have to go to the emergency room, right away!" he almost yelled.

"Oh, fuck the emergency room. I'm going on holiday in three days..."

"Man, with those symptoms they'll take you out of turn! I know what I'm talking about. A few years ago my arm went dead and they took me immediately out of turn, although the waiting room was full. It turned out to be a nerve. But you are much worse. You can't feel half your body and you can't hear."

Male friendships. After female friendships, male friendships are the second sleaziest human relationships in the universe. A few years ago Boro's work broke him down into a bunch of symptoms, and I begged him to go to the doctor's. Now it was my

Tomislav Birtić

turn. He begged me to get in a taxi right away, that very second, and go to the emergency room.

"OK, since you insist, I'll go by bus, have a shower at home, then I'll go to the emergency room."

"What are you talking about? In your state, in this heat, by bus!? You are going by taxi! Now!"

"OK, I will do what you say and go to the emergency room, I am going, but just don't make a bigger drama out of it than it really is. I am going by bus."

I could tell by his face that he was thinking about the situation. He would rather I went by taxi, but he was afraid that if he insisted on a taxi I might not go to the doctor's at all, having had a hard time persuading me, so he unwillingly agreed to me going by bus.

I packed up my things, loaded my back-pack onto my back, and set off to the bus stop. In less than five minutes he was on the phone.

"Listen, don't have a shower. Please, I really mean this. I don't want you on my conscience. Smell as bad as you like, but don't go home. Go straight to the emergency room."

"Alright then. I wouldn't give in to your taxi idea, so whatever, I won't go home, but I will go straight to the doctor's."

What can I say... Over the past few weeks, as it got worse and worse, I had been getting worried. Now I was just scared. I was really scared. After I told the doctors my symptoms, in the packed waiting room, they sent me out of turn to the neurologist... that was real fear. The waiting room was full of all kinds of people, from children to old men who could barely sit, and I, a young looking old horse, in front of all those unhappy and reproachful eyes, was sent in to a doctor, as though I had pulled some strings. But my only strings were in fact – my symptoms.

To cut a long story short, the neurologist, using the very basic tests, like the police use to see if a driver is drunk (walking a straight line, closing your eyes and touching your ear with your left hand...) excluded a stroke. But, he told me that if I go on living such an unhealthy life, which I described to him in detail during the examination, I would certainly suffer the consequences. I would wake up at about seven. Before I got out of bed, I would light a cigarette. Sometimes I would not get up until after my third, and I would smoke another three or four with coffee (I was a chain smoker, I would smoke three to, in the most stressful days or when I was on duty, five packets of strong cigarettes a day). I didn't eat breakfast. At work I would drink more coffee, and for my first meal – depending on the day, depending on my work, between noon and two o'clock – I would get something delivered. We were so busy that we didn't go out for a lunch break, we didn't even have a canteen, so we only ate food we could get delivered. It was mainly fried meat and fried potatoes. If it was the first meat fried in the same oil, it was still edible, but more often it was somewhere between more brown and black than yellow and brown; empty calories. I would occasionally order beans with sausage, pizza or pasta. Whatever I ate, I would drink a lot of Coca Cola, and when I got hungry again after lunch, I would eat a Snickers bar from the coin machine (or Twix or Bounty), or I would order a sandwich from Subway, because it was a five minute drive from the office, so the delivery came very quickly. At about six p.m. I would set off for home. By bus, then tram.

Tomislav Birtić

I would pop into my local café and drink sometimes two or three, more often five or six beers. In the shop at the bottom of the building where I lived I would sometimes buy a two-litre bottle of Coca Cola, to wash my mouth out from the cigarettes I had long since stopped enjoying. I would often buy two or three chocolate bars with the cigarettes and soda, again Snickers, Bounty, Twix, which I would start eating in the lift. Sometimes at eight, or sometimes after ten in the evening I would fry myself an egg and ham, bacon or cheese, or eggs with bacon and cheese, or I would make myself a serious sandwich with all imaginable spreads, ham, cheese, and I would eat it, staring at the television, until I was overcome by sleep. And so it went on, day after day, and at the weekends too.

The neurologist sent me for an ECG. After the test I was taken over by an experienced doctor, who was teaching a student or a new colleague. I told her too, in detail, just as I had the neurologist, everything I was doing to destroy myself, while I was still alive. It turned out that for a smoker who smoked at least three packets a day, and who ate exclusively fat and chocolate, I had an incredibly healthy heart, and lungs. But, the experienced doctor, whatever her specialization was, was also a specialist in psychology...

"So, every man's dream, to be surrounded, half naked, by two women," she said to me.

"You could have given me a general anaesthetic before you said that," I laughed.

It was a tragic scene. A sweaty fatso, sweating from the summer heat and fear, my stomach tumbling deep below my belt, surrounded by two good-looking lady doctors, and the awareness that there was no point in asking even an average woman out for coffee – let alone – if I could choose this is what I would choose – the more experienced, who was also the better looking one of the two.

"Mr. Birtić, this time you have been lucky. False alarm. That is, the final warning for your body. But, if you go on doing what you have been doing for years, you will come to see us again, but next time you will not be going home," said the lady doctor. "You need to stop smoking, but I don't expect you to do what I say. That is why you need to lose weight. You really must. You have no choice. You will either lose weight or the results could be disastrous."

"Can I go on holiday, or would retirement be a better idea?"

"You joke. But, as I said, lose weight!"

On 27th July 2006 (I remember the date from the photograph my love of that time sent to DeviantArt) I left the emergency room with all the symptoms I had come there with, weighing 295 pounds (134 kilos), but as light as a feather. I am not going to die, I am not in mortal danger.

A MANAGER'S ANNUAL LEAVE

I arrived at the coast with the firm intention of swimming at least a half mile (a little more than one kilometre) every morning and evening. Almost nul points.

For the first few days I woke up at about noon, and I counted it as a success if I managed to make myself get out of bed and move on to the balcony, where I would sit and surf the web. I was in no mood or condition to go swimming. In the evening I made myself go into the water, but I would get tired after just a few minutes. I was not able to swim even thirty meters in one go. I would float on the water for a while, and then I would come out of the water. I would cover the three hundred or so meters, gently uphill, with a thirty meter difference in altitude from the beach to the apartment, by stopping several times for a minute or two. Climbing back up to the apartment caused me such physical and mental effort, that I had no desire to go down to the beach.

Half way through my holiday, at the end of the first week, I felt as though my arms and legs and half my head were less wooden, and my hearing was slowly coming back. I still could not take a deep breath, but at least I had no more pain in my chest.

When I went back to work, I could hear in both ears, and the woodenness had almost completely gone. But, you could have said anything to me, just not that I needed to lose weight. My parents and sister tried, and I reacted very irritably.

"SON, DO YOU KNOW ANYONE WHO WALKS EVERYWHERE WHO IS FAT?"

Not long after I got back from my holiday I had a nervous breakdown. The third in ten years.

I woke up at about noon. Instead of being shocked because I had slept for most of my working day, I just lay there, staring at the ceiling. I wanted my boss to tell me it would be best for me to leave the firm. To fire me. Or for him to advise me to change my job.

I lay there for about half an hour. He called. I didn't answer the phone. I looked at my missed calls, of course he called several times.

Somehow I made myself get dressed and set out to the office. He called again, but I still didn't answer. One minute to the office I sent him a message. To be my boss and my friend and to come down to the café across the road from the office. That is what happened.

He said hello. I didn't. If I had said a word, I would have started wailing. Which would have been embarrassing in a café full of my colleagues. For a while both of us were silent.

"Have you had lunch?" I asked him. A tear slid down below my sunglasses.

"No."

"Then go and get something to eat, and when you get back I will have sorted myself out".

Just as he should have, to avoid an explosion, he went without a word. And, what was very important, he didn't touch me. No tap on the shoulder, no manly hitting fist on fist. Precisely what was needed.

He came back, and I had sorted myself out sufficiently to be able to listen. That is, to listen and understand. So that I actually knew what he was talking about.

"Look," Boris began, "you would probably most like to quit, but it would be a big relief if I fired you."

"Oh yes."

"Unfortunately, it's not going to happen. I need you."

"Fuck!"

One or two syllables was the right amount. A third would have made me cry.

"What is happening to you is classic burn out. A textbook case. And, what are friends for, but to make things worse. I have gone through it twice and both times I solved the problem by changing my job. That would be the best for you too. But I need you. I respect any decision you make, but I want you here."

"OK."

"Hold on just a few more months, and then we will see. Either we will reduce your work load, or give you a new job description, we will think of something..."

"OK."

He went back to work, and I went to get a bus. I didn't change to a tram as usual, but I walked to the embankment; Zagreb has a lovely path along the river. I barely managed to walk one kilometre. Wet through, struggling to breathe, I sat on a bench to have a rest. Well, at least that was something, I finally managed to take a deep breath.

I sat and thought. I tried to remember the last time I had played any sport. Years and years ago. Up until my sixth birthday I lived in the country, where children play outside all day long, eat like wolves and are still skinny. When I was ten I started to play tennis, and later all day long between training sessions for high jump, I would play football and basketball, and somewhat less volleyball and table tennis, right up until I went to university. Then came the three hungry years of the war, and in 1992, as thin as a rake from malnutrition, I started work as a sports writer. Amongst other things, I covered volleyball. Getting better, putting on some weight, I played tennis with volleyball players, which came to an end when they left Mladost to go abroad, and due to my frequent travel, in 1996. That was when I started to go downhill. Work, out for drinks after work, bad food. Gradually, from 154 pounds (70 kilos), my weight rose to 295 (134). This was, by all accounts, either the end of my weakness, or the end of me. Now I needed to do something with myself, or I would cease to be.

My old man had told me a million times. "Son, do you know anyone who is fat who walks everywhere?" Aware that I was too fat to run, that my ankles, knees and hips and spine would not survive running, trying to persuade me to save myself, he told me about waiters and waitresses who do not carry heavy weights, but since as they work they walk all the time, they are all skinny (that is, the percentage of slim waiters is so high that we can say that they are all slim), about friends and acquaintances for whom walking was their only recreation, and they looked great. For years he had given me advice, talked, almost begged me to save myself, scaring me with what would happen.

That day, on the way to my flat, I didn't buy any chocolate, or beer, nothing fattening. But tomatoes and mozzarella cheese, and apples.

Tomislav Birtić

THREE UNSUCCESSFUL ATTEMPTS TO LOSE WEIGHT, BY THE BOOK. NO. 1 MAGIC CELERIAC SOUP

Of course on the road from 155 to 295 pounds (70 to 134 kilos), I had tried several times to lose weight by starving myself.

The first diet was recommended by Nedjeljko Šević, known as Beg, a colleague who had done the layout for two of my books. I called into his studio and was amazed to see that he was half the man he had been. I asked him how he had done it. "You won't be hungry, and you will lose weight," he encouraged me. "It's a magic soup based on celeriac, which I think removes all the water, and it really works. So, you can eat the soup whenever you want and as much as you want, once a week you treat yourself to a medium sized steak, with tomatoes, and bananas. You can only drink coffee with no sugar."

He gave me the recipe. Boil a head of savoy cabbage, a kilo of celeriac root, two peppers, three onions or leaks, a litre of tomato puree, two bouillon cubes. That was it. You could eat that soup as much as you wanted, whenever you wanted. If I felt like eating at midnight, at three in the morning, no problem, literally whenever I wanted. But I was not allowed to eat anything else, except on the fourth day I was allowed to eat a steak or some kind of beef, no more than a quarter of a kilo, and with it I was allowed to eat six tomatoes. On the fifth day I was allowed to eat three bananas.

And really, the pounds (kilos) came off, it was amazing. But. But, as soon as I had eaten two good meals, my weight returned.

"ADMIT IT, YOU WOULD KILL FOR A PIECE OF MEAT RIGHT NOW". THE DIET OF THE WORLD CUP 1998 BRONZE MEDAL WINNERS DIDN'T HELP EITHER

While I was still eating the magic soup, which, although I lost 8 pounds (4 kilos) a week, made me feel sick after a month (I got nauseous just looking at it), I was recommended to try another diet by the then president of the Croatian Football Federation, Vlatko Marković.

"Admit it, you would kill for a piece of meat right now," Marković said to me at that time.

"Yes. How to put it, if it wouldn't kill me, I would kill for a piece of meat," I joked.

"Well, now I will tell you about the diet that has bought me a lot of drinks from our national football team..." Don't forget that that was the team that came third in the World Cup in 1998, and included Champions' League winners, respectable German league players, demi-gods from Series A, the best paid in the world...

He took a piece of paper and quickly wrote out a menu for an entire week, day by day. So, the first day, grilled meat, the second day, boiled meat, the third day, green salad with boiled egg, the fourth day fish, and so on, up to the seventh day – just meat. This diet also worked while I stuck to it, but the weight came back as soon as I had eaten two normal meals. I thought, I suppose all this starvation makes sense if you need to lose a couple of pounds (kilo) you have put on, or you haven't lost any weight for a while by exercising, or you have eaten more than you lost by exercising. So all you need to do is to get yourself in order. That diet solves all the problems of sportsmen, but not us office types.

AND THEN I GOT IT: THE PROBLEM SUGGESTS ITS OWN SOLUTION. STARVATION SUGGESTS MOVEMENT

The third recipe for slimming was dictated to me by the good angel of our neighbourhood, Puška (Rifle), a true sportsman in body and mind, a good restaurant owner, a better cook, and an even better human being. Listening to his advice, I did not mix proteins and carbohydrates, I did not eat after seven in the evening (or some days after eight), and if I really did want a pizza, then pizza would be all I ate that day. Then the same thing happened. If you don't stick to the asceticism for two days, the weight returns...

I tried to trick nature using diets without exercising. The problem suggests its own solution. Exercise!

A couple of times I bought a variety of pieces of exercise apparatus, from television ads. With the excuse that it was banging on my parquet floor, and the noise was annoying the neighbours, I gave my abs workout apparatus to my friend three days after I had bought it. It was huge, it just got in the way in my already over-crowded studio apartment. I also bought an exercise bike, and for a while I would watch matches riding it, and not sitting or lying down. The bike even served for a while as a clothes horse, but I gave it away in the end as well. To my sister. I also tried some slimming pills. They only helped me in the morning, because as soon as I took them in the morning I would run to the toilet...

But this time it was different. Really different. Just as the Ode to Joy appears in the Ninth Symphony only as a hint of victory, so, despite my demotivating, depressing fatigue after walking less than a kilometre, this sentence finally broke through to my consciousness: "Son, do you know anyone who walks everywhere who is fat?" I decided, but this time I firmly decided, to walk as much as I could. That is, according to the rules of recreational sport. If I could only walk five meters, I would walk five meters and rest. And then another five meters! I would get my organism used to increasing effort, so we would see what would happen, what would come of it.

Tomislav Birtić

THE MIRROR IS LYING, AND PERHAPS THE SCALES AS WELL, BUT THE BELT IS SURELY TELLING THE TRUTH

Let me tell you what you really want to know. I lost 59 pounds (27 kilos) in four months.

For the first month I didn't dare weigh myself. Like a soldier counting the days until the end of his military service – he won't start on the first day. Why? To get on the scales and see that I no longer weighed 295 but 294 or 293 pounds? Just as depressing. And those scales... You never know what their degree of error is. How can scales that cost ten or thirty bucks be accurate? No way!

The mirror is another enemy. First because your reflection in it is true, and then because your reflection is an optical illusion. No joke. At the beginning of my dieting I was really fat. Absolutely, simply, fat. However, as I lost weight, I seemed to look fatter and fatter. The flab first of all disappeared from the places where it had formed last – my face. That is what I noticed after a week and a half. Super. Then I lost weight from my legs, so I looked like a barrel standing on toothpicks.

But the barrel is another story. I lost flab from it layer by layer. First from my chest, so my stomach was nicely emphasized. My belly, and the fat on my hips. Then it seemed as though the fat was being taken off by someone scraping with a shovel, heaps of fat falling off my hips. Which only served to emphasize my stomach. In the final phase the layer of fat on my stomach would also disappear.

And so, round and round. As the next layer came off my chest, my stomach would again look bigger than it really was. I took a layer off my hips, and my stomach looked even bigger, and so on and so on.

So I believed my belt, and I lived for the morning when my trousers would have fallen down if I hadn't made a new hole in my belt. I needed a new hole in my belt in a month.

I only weighed myself after I had to make a new hole in my belt. After the fourth hole I didn't shout for joy, I didn't shed a tear, but I expressed all my excitement to myself: 235 pounds!! (107 kilos). Wow, 59 pounds (27 kilos) less in only four months.

This is how.

I PERFECTED THE BOLLETTIERI METHOD

For four months I skipped breakfast, for lunch I ate a tomato and mozzarella cheese, and for supper an apple with Emmentaler cheese, or an apple with prosciutto ham, always with a glass of red wine. A glass is one decilitre. I stopped drinking beer. I didn't give up alcohol, but when I was with friends I drank red wine with water (in Croatia we call it Bevanda). I didn't even hold back, I never missed a round, I would drink five or six Bevandas with my friends, but I wouldn't drink more than one glass when I was at home. In four months I didn't eat a single cake, not a single piece of chocolate, not a gram of bread (at the party in our office to celebrate the birth of my colleague's baby, I took just two slices of ham and the same amount of cheese, so as not to spoil the fun). And I walked.

I read that the great tennis coach Nick Bollettieri said: "Never lose three times in a row. If you lose twice, find an absolute beginner and thrash him. You will feel better." I don't know if he really said that, or someone published those words because it sounded good. But... Coach, when I was looking for Mirjana Lučić in New York, you did not give me a statement, but thank you for this from the bottom of my heart. It is a great, great thought. I had quoted that sentence countless times, but this time I decided to apply the advice. Not exactly literally, but almost literally, dead tired after walking a kilometre I remembered Nick once again. For year and years I had been losing, not able to find an absolute beginner to thrash to death and feel better. I dragged myself home, lay down on the couch, stared at the ceiling for a while and made a vow. Not after two defeats in a row, but every day, I would find an opponent to trash and so feel better. Of course, I meant myself.

I was my own opponent, made to measure.

I was surprised that already after a week and a half I was able to walk about a little less than two miles (three kilometres) without a break. At the end of the first month, I was encouraged enough to walk home from the office – about five miles (eight kilometres). I made a deal with myself that I would walk as much as I could, and then get on a bus, or, depending where I was overtaken by tiredness, call a taxi. I was more than pleasantly surprised when I walked the entire distance from work to home, without a break.

I started going home from work on foot every day.

And even further... Further was pure poetry.

Tomislav Birtić

WHAT IS TIME?
OR: EXERCISE CONQUERS STRESS

"Have you lost weight?" a top manager asked me, no matter who, no matter in what field he works, when he saw me a month after I had started walking.

Oh dear, I had slimmed down one hole (a huge hole!) on my belt, but I was so fat that the slimming was not obvious...

"Oh yes," I managed to say, happily, "one hole on my belt."

"How? Do you run? Running did it for me."

He was always careful about what he ate. And he was also careful about what he drank – often only water – let alone what he ate. The few healthy meals I had eaten in the years when I was gaining weight I ate with him. Lean meat, mainly turkey or veal, with salad, or fresh (cottage) cheese with salad. The most unhealthy thing he ate with me, but only once or twice, was a Margherita pizza. Of course, it was a small one, with water. I don't ever remember seeing him eat anything sweet. He was also under a great deal of stress. A hundred or so telephone calls every day, hundreds of thousands of miles behind the wheel, days, weeks and months at airports and in aeroplanes...

Fortunately, a friend of his family was a psychologist. She told him that his only problem was stress, and the cure for it was physical activity. That top manager, now and then, let's say on average once a week, played football with his childhood friends. We know how that works. The hardest thing in the world is to find a partner for bridge. Football? Too many people to find. The psychologist recommended running. She to him, him to me.

"Unfortunately, I am afraid my joints are no good, they wouldn't stand running. I walk, and I eat only tomatoes with mozzarella for lunch and apples with a little ham for supper. Sometimes the other way round," I laughed.

"Well, if walking helps you, just you walk," my friend said. "Since I've been running, there isn't much that can upset me..."

Well, yes, I knew exactly what he was talking about.

In the first week of walking I already noticed that I was not so irritable any more. I would like to say, one of the most frequent excuses given by people who do not exercise is the desire to spend as much time as possible with their family. But, what actually is "time"? Is it three hours lying on the couch and yelling at any squeak, complaining to the wife because her hair is behind and not over her ears, and what are the slippers doing to the left instead of to the right of the armchair, or is it two hours after exercise, and in those two hours nothing bothers you, you have patience for your wife and children, and absolutely nothing can throw you off balance? That's my point! The stress at work was the same, but I was not the same. There was nothing I would react to irritably, offensively.

THE ENTIRE STADIUM STOOD UP
AND APPLAUDED ME

The marathon taught me that you can earn an ovation either by beating everyone else, or by beating yourself. In the very civilized Scandinavian countries, the crowd stands up often to congratulate marathon runners, regardless where they are placed, but otherwise they only show respect in that way to the medal winners – and the fighters who enter the stadium last, perhaps four hours after the winner.

In my second month of walking, I dared to walk all around a lake, Jarun. For a beginner, it was like Colombo setting off to sail the Atlantic. I had no idea how many miles it was, nor how my body would take it. Hm, it didn't. Somewhere about half way round, my legs were like lead. My steps were short, I pushed myself, but I would not allow myself to sit and have a rest.

At the end of the path I felt like a marathon runner probably feels when he comes into the stadium, glorifying in the applause of the crowd. Yes, the entire stadium stood up and congratulated me with their applause and deafening ovation, for conquering myself. It did not. But it felt like it did.

I had an apple and a bit of ham for supper, I drank a glass of red wine, and I felt like the king of the world. Actually, not "like". I was the king of the world, and to be the king of my own life, the exterminator of my own weaknesses, was all I needed that evening and not only that evening, to be truly king of the world. Until then I had been convinced, but from that evening I was sure, that the arrow had been released and was flying towards it target, that the flab had received its sentence and the sentence was irrevocable. An amazingly good feeling.

SO THEY WOULDN'T HAVE TO AIR
THE OFFICE AFTER ME

I came into my brokers' office... and I wish they had had a carpet and not parquet floors. The sweat was dripping, dripping, dripping off me, forming a puddle at my feet the size of a postcard, then A4 paper... The drips were splashing off the floor up to somewhere below my knees. I sat down in an armchair being careful not to lean back, because after I took my rucksack off, my back was soaked.

"Oh OK Tom, last time you visited we had to air the office for two days after you left, and now you have destroyed our parquet and the entire furnishings," said the analyst. He said it seriously, trying to make it sound like a joke, but the others were falling about laughing at the scene.

"OK, OK, I'll change my perfume," I also tried hard to sound like I was joking.

"..."

It seems I said it too seriously, and financiers tend to take things literally.

"I get it, I get it..." I assured them.

Joking aside, I walked everywhere. Sometimes I would get on a bus or tram, but I could no longer stand the crowds, nor waiting at traffic lights. In a bus or tram I felt like I was in chains, completely helpless. I would hold out for two stops, get off and enjoy the freedom of the open air. Simply, I would leave early enough to make my appointments. In just a few weeks, I had measured and timed all the routes I took, and I would arrive right on time, to the minute, or a little too early.

The problem was that the result of all that walking was the increasing power of my organism. You don't even notice how fast you are walking. I didn't even sweat at all, until I stopped. And then the sweat would just pour out of me.

As a compromise, for meetings where I was not permitted to smell, I would take a taxi or a tram, but wherever I could, I would walk.

THE DOORMAN KNOWS
WHO THE IDIOT IN THE RAIN IS

I introduced a rule. No excuse! No excuse!

We all know how that goes. I am busy today, so I won't walk. It's raining, so I won't walk. I have to go to someone's birthday, I'll skip my exercise today. Oh no! I walked even if axes were falling from the sky. OK, axes never actually fell, but nothing could stop me. If it was time for me to go home from work, and it was raining, I would walk from the office to my flat holding an umbrella. On the bridge the cars would drive through puddles and splash me, drench me with water, but I had a higher goal, my health. Plus, consistent as I was, I became greater in my own eyes. I was greater in the eyes of my colleagues at work, who wanted to give me a lift, but I would say thank you and refuse. I enjoyed the compliments to my determination.

If I was at meetings all day, where I was not allowed to be sweaty, I would walk around my neighbourhood, even as late as ten or eleven at night.

If it was too muddy on the embankment or the path, to avoid walking in the mud, I would take a bus or tram from work to where I live, then I would walk around the athletics track. There is a paved path around it. Holding my umbrella, up to twenty circuits. On the first day the doorman at the swimming pool, which is right next to the stadium, came out and gave me a funny look. For a few of my circuits he stood at the door, watching me, and it seemed he was about to ask me what I was doing, but he didn't drive me away. He saw that I wasn't causing any problems, so he let me be.

I would also go there on days when there was a storm brewing. I would start to walk, and if the weather held out, it wouldn't catch me half way round the lake, where I had nowhere to shelter. Here I had somewhere to run, into the café at the swimming pool.

Tomislav Birtić

A NEW WORLD – A BRAVE NEW WORLD!

Going on foot, or, to flatter myself by raising myself to the level of a sportsman, race walking, I discovered a better world, free of cynicism, nihilism, a world which welcomes a novice, wishing him all the best, cheering him on. It is no exaggeration to say, a world that celebrates life and not death, victory and not defeat.

You know, the crowd from the café are not a bad lot. They are just the majority. At work or in the café, they are the same, good people. But, it is hard to get up from the table and leave; it is hard not to drink one more round, even if it is too much; it is hard to overcome yourself. And because it is so hard, if someone decides to stop smoking, or lose weight, instead of encouragement, he gets "Aaaaa, I wonder how long it's going to last this time!" He gets a back-drop of noise, like in a quiz when someone gives the wrong answer. It is crazy how many societies glorify getting drunk, over-eating, self-destruction and deca-dence of all kinds, and how part of that celebration is a bad attitude towards someone else's redemption, camouflaged as an equally bad joke.

The beneficial effects of small changes are highly praised in lay psychology. A weekend at the sea, an outing, any kind of change for the better... However, not even one mile or just one kilometre from the local café, or the café where I used to sit with my colleagues after work, I discovered a completely new world. It was the world of overcoming oneself. An army of sisters and brothers active in their decision to align themselves with nature, and to offer one another support. In our healthy routines on the paths to health, we get to know one another without a word, with no impolite comments on who is losing weight more quickly, who looks better, whose smile is happier, we greet each other in passing, waving our hands in greeting or giving a thumbs up... I don't know any names, but we are sisters and brothers in our decision, optimism, and finally in our victory. Victory becomes completely normal in time. It becomes usual. All of a sudden victory is no longer something to celebrate. Some say "a normal day in the office," but for us a normal day on the embankment was in fact a normal day, in harmony with nature. It was added value in life.

From the very first, we were sisters and brothers in discipline – discipline assumes action against your own will – and then in enjoyment. Yes, at the beginning of change there was discipline. I walked, I was careful what, how much and when I ate. However, from the mantra of walking and careful eating the will for life was born. And just as money sticks to money, so the will for life sticks to the will for life. Then the will for life starts to grow, and grow, to flare up, and you have the feeling you could tunnel through a mountain. The closer you are to your image of yourself, the closer you have brought your imagination to reality, the more will you have, and you become addicted to exercise.

Overcoming the routine of work, home and café, launching out into liberation, I discovered my city for a second time. T'ai chi practitioners, people medi-

Tomislav Birtić

tating, people who love their dogs, fathers kicking a ball about with their children, people throwing Frisbees, playing badminton, all of this exists in my city. And I am with them.

"MY FRIEND, YOU DON'T SMELL ANY MORE!"

Hm, you are what you eat, what you carry inside you, what you do, what you... this and that... let's say that this is dubious. But I have absolutely no doubt that you smell of what you eat. Or, at the very least, since my friend and colleague Stjepan Banović said enthusiastically, "My friend, you don't smell anymore! Since you have started eating healthy food your smell has changed," no one can persuade me that our smell does not depend on the number of schnitzels that were previously fried in the oil in which the schnitzel was fried that they have delivered to you.

For people who do not have the privilege of being brutally honest with someone, my conversations with my friends look like arguments. To joke a little, it does have its good side. I will allow myself to be a friend to everyone: If you eat disgusting food, and no one has told you that your smell is not a matter of taking a shower or perfume, it is perhaps because you do not have a friend like my Stjepan. Smile!

Tomislav Birtić

I CAN STAND UP WITHOUT SUPPORTING MYSELF WITH MY HANDS ON THE CHAIR

When I was fat, I would get up from a couch or chair, at least according to the older generation, like the goal keeper Lav Jashin after he threw himself at a ball – it would take me half an hour. I was sluggish, my knees could not take my weight, so I would stand up, supporting myself with both hands on the arms of the chair or couch, like an old man with a stick.

The change for the better was as much a surprise to me as to the people who cared. My parents came to visit me. My mum wanted to get up and fetch something from the kitchen. In the bad old days, I would have a hard time overtaking her, that is, I would get up quicker than her, but only by an inch. This time, she didn't manage to move at all, to her and my dad's delighted amazement, I flew off the couch like a sprinter out of the starting blocks.

Although progress must by its nature be gradual, and it is, a noticeable change is always surprising. Nothing happens overnight, but it seems just as if it did, as if it was overnight. In the evening everything is just as it was the day before, but in the morning your trousers fall down if you don't punch another hole in your belt. Yesterday you got up from your chair by supporting yourself with your hands, today it is like you were flung from a catapult.

WHAT A DISGRACE – AN EXECUTIVE EDITOR – WALKING

Every so often a little devil with a trident on your shoulder whispers to you to give up. To surrender.

My mobile rang, just half way across the bridge.

"So, you really are walking?!" the head of the brokers' house said in honest amazement.

"What kind of question is that?"

"I thought you were having us on."

"I don't understand."

"Well, the whole time I was thinking you were joking, that everyone at work was pulling my leg – telling me you walk everywhere, until right now, until I saw you from my car, saw you with my own eyes, I didn't believe either you or them. OK – I saw you in town. He drove himself here, parked.... But half way across the bridge! You really aren't lying. You really are walking."

"There you are."

"Come on, please, drive. As soon as I get to work I will tell the guys that we can have a whip round and buy you a car. What will our other clients think of us if they see you walking? What kind of investment bankers are we? Who will believe us if we are not able to take care of the executive editor of internationaly awarded 24sata?" he laughed. "If we have driven you to ruin, if you don't have enough to take a tram, let alone a car, what is in store for those mere mortals... It's boiling hot. You can fry an egg on the car body, the tarmac is red hot, and you are walking! It's pouring with rain, you are walking..."

"Well you can tell your clients who ask about my walking that I am an eccentric. Tell them, Tom has flipped his lid. Or, if nothing else helps, tell them the truth," even I burst out laughing, "that I ended up in the emergency room so now I have to walk."

"If you don't care about us any more, think about the reputation of your own company. The executive editor of 24sata doesn't drive, he goes on foot. Who in his right mind will want to work for you if even the second man on the paper doesn't have enough for a car?" he was killing himself laughing...

"He-he, I am not the only second man there. The first man and the other "second men" drive dangerous machines. There are enough of those who worry about the reputation of the company."

The director of my brokers was not the only one to say, "The executive editor of 24sata – walking!" Some of my business partners joked that they would send me a driver, not for my sake, but so they would not have the embarrassment of meeting with a pedestrian. Some of them meant it seriously.

But, my doctors also meant it seriously. Me too. With unconcealed delight, I was burning up my flab. Being in the centre of attention did not bother me at all. On the contrary. I was succeeding in what many others can only dream about.

WOW! EVERYTHING LOOKS GOOD ON ME

Putting on weight is like one of those wars where no one knows any more who started it, whose fault it was, but everyone knows the number of casualties. If you wake up and you don't fit in your trousers, you can't do up the last button on your shirt... Instead of waking up as soon as I became too big for my clothes, I simply bought new ones. I hid my stomach under a waistcoat with hundreds of pockets, which I wore even in unbearable heat. I probably let my hair grow long unconsciously, so my bulldog, or boxer cheeks wouldn't stand out so much. Yeah right.

As I lost weight, my old clothes began to suit me again and my new shirts looked like dresses on me. Almost an inch (two centimetres) from my neck to my collar. A sweet chasm. Not aesthetic, but so aesthetic. A fashion crime which even the god of design would forgive. However, I was never so happy in a shop as when I went to find a jacket. For years I had chosen on the basis of a single criterion, that is concealing my belly as much as possible. I will never forget how I tried on several models that day, and they all looked good on me. It didn't matter that they didn't have my size. I am after all two meters tall with long arms. A beautiful flat surface, not a pear-shaped protuberance, but a flat surface stretched down from my neck to below my belt...

Tomislav Birtić

PROGRESS IS AN INEXHAUSTIBLE
SOURCE OF DETERMINATION

Now we have reached February 2007. Of course I wasn't hungry that night. But I wanted something that makes you fat. Pizza, lasagne, steak, pancakes with a finger thick spread, anything sweet... Or I wanted to reward myself by any form of decadence. Something like a Chicago celebration with a cigar, in a public place, precisely in Utah, where the legislation is rigorous.

I told myself, I will weigh myself, so if I still weigh 235 pounds (107 kilos), the only thing for it is to decide what I will eat. I got on the scales, and whoopee! 229 pounds! (104 kilos). So I decided to celebrate my progress with an apple.

And truly, it is true for both competitive sportsmen and for recreational sportsmen, and those who are convalescing – progress gives you strength. There is nothing a sportsman won't put up with, no demands from his coach he won't meet, if he is convinced that the method is producing excellent results. If I had weighed 235 pounds that night, that is 60 less than at the beginning of the story, my fall would have lasted for one single meal, I would have eaten some meat with potatoes or noodles, but as it was, at 6 pounds (3 kilos) less than the last time I had weighed myself, 66 less than on my first day of dieting. No way! I thought, nothing is going to stop me going below 220 pounds (100 kilos).

To show that this is no fairy tale, I will soon be writing about problems.

That is, a bit more excitement, the climax of the fairy tale, then problems.

oooooooooooo!

Right on the threshold of the office, Boris, Renato and Zoran, the three from the beginning of the book, from the episode about going to the emergency room, treated me to an ""Ooooooooooooooooo!"

I stopped, looked myself over, theatrically, from my feet to my chin, and stood in a pose of wonderment, with my arms bent at the elbows and palms turned towards them.

"Today you look.... classy," said Boris.

Actually I looked like I did many other days. Khaki corduroy trousers, with a slim pullover with wide horizontal stripes, white tennis shoes. Like many other days, but not quite completely the same. I weighed 66 pounds (30 kilos) less than many days when I did not deserve a fanfare when I walked into the office. The fanfare lacked an addition – that is the entire greeting, with the unexpressed addition, should have been: "Ooooooooooooooooo! You are no longer hiding your flab under jumpers and photographer's waistcoats, but you are wearing that tight sweater. You are simply slim!"

That is why it is worth losing weight.

VICTORY!!! NAPKIN ON MY LAP!

I can't explain why, but when I was fat I was never able to tuck a napkin into my collar. Perhaps because the angle, falling from my neck down under the table, only served to highlight my stomach A fat, fleshy head over two dark oil stains or whatever on a white napkin. If the napkins aren't white, they are certainly in some other treacherous colour, which dominates the restaurant amongst the dark suits or other clothes. And now, if a little food falls on a dark shirt, it is easier to deal with than my belly, overemphasized by a clean and unstained napkin.

Putting the napkin on my knees made no sense. That is, somehow I managed to get it under my belly, and from above I could see maybe a half of inch (centimetre of two) of napkin. It was an art to miss my stomach and hit the barely visible ribbon of napkin unconcealed by my flab with the food.

So for many years my napkin remained on the table.

About half a year after the beginning of my slimming campaign, I went to lunch with my investment banker. There are no words to describe the feeling when I triumphantly placed the napkin on my knees. What a beautiful rectangle, what a wonderful triumphant view, that immense expanse of napkin spread over my knees.

Tomislav Birtić

"WOW, TOM, ALL THE GIRLS ARE TALKING ABOUT YOU!"

Everyone is watching everything. Everyone is watching everything about everyone, on everyone. A man is made by his clothes, a man is made by his salary, he is made by what take out he orders, his cell phone, the drink he orders in a café, the flowers he sends or does not send, and to whom he sends them or does not send them, his watch, the number of conversation he has with his boss in a unit of time... There is an endless list of things which it is humanly and politically correct to say do not make a man, but at the end of the day a man is in fact made by them.

Finally, it is man that makes man like that, defined by the criteria of the World Health Organization, and by the criteria of men's and women's magazines, advertisements for all that apparatus and preparations from telemarketing. We are all part of the saying, "I have seen better, I have slept with worse," and we all want to have the best position possible in that joke. We all know how we would like to look, we all see in the mirror and in other people's eyes how we look and, apart from those who are so self-aware that they don't need a compliment, we seek confirmation from others that we are the same, or at least as similar to ourselves as we imagine ourselves to be.

The belt had long since been telling me what I wanted to hear, I conquered miles and miles with ever increasing ease, and ever increasing enjoyment, and the scales told the same story. The cream on the top was when my colleague Renato, who came into the office as though he had hardly waited to reach the assistant head's office, across the meters and meters of our office, to tell the joyful news: "Wow, Tom, all the girls are talking about you!"

It's true! We are all so self-confident, our looks don't matter, the appearance of a man does not make the man, and we don't care. But in the life of every former fatso there is a Renato, who will tell him that all the girls in the office are talking about him. If he deserves to hear that.

Tomislav Birtić

THE BEST 5 KILOMETRES
AT 7 KM AN HOUR

I introduce Zijo, that is Dr. Zijad Duraković, to everyone as Tuđman's doctor from the time when Croatian president Tuđman was healthy. When I was running some errands in the city centre, I ran into Zijo. He, as is appropriate for a doctor, immediately noticed that I had visibly lost weight.

"Sixty six pounds!" I boasted.

"In how much time?"

"In four and a half months. Maybe five months."

"Uh, maybe that is a bit too quick. But for now, let's just say that it is a wonderful success. May I ask how you lost weight?"

"Every day I walk at least ten kilometres (six miles), I don't mixed proteins and carbohydrates, that means I eat a tomato and mozzarella or an apple and ham, and after six or seven in the evening I only eat fruit, or maybe a slice of Emmenthaler."

"Excellent! Well done!"

We hadn't seen each other in a long time, so we made use of this chance meeting to have a cup of coffee. Again, as is appropriate for a doctor, Zijo appealed to me to stop smoking.

"And listen, managers like you often don't have time for exercise, or they make the excuse of having no time. But you are doing great, it would be a shame to give up. So, if you don't have time to do ten kilometres, walk five kilometres at seven kilometres an hour. That is really healthy."

NORDIC WALKING POLES, THE BEST INVESTMENT IN HEALTH OF ALL TIME, AND AN EPIC DISCOVERY OF MUSCLES

I saw several walkers on the embankment using poles. Most of them were as slim as marathon runners, and all of them had better posture than I did. They were as straight as if they had swallowed a broom. The only difference between them was how they reacted to the gaze of interested people like me. Some were bothered by it.

From an article published in the magazine Lider, I learned that it is called Nordic walking, that using that method of walking, you use 46 per cent more energy, and that Nordic walking poles could be purchased in Rost Šport by the Dom sportova in Zagreb.

Various sources mainly agree that Nordic walking makes you use 90 per cent of your muscles, and one hour Nordic walking burns up to 500 calories, about 40 per cent more than walking without poles. Nordic walking preserves your ankles, knees and back, Nordic walking strengthens your heart, your pulse rate is about 15 per cent faster...

Whatever the case, I resisted for a long time, but then one Sunday in my fourth month of walking, I covered twenty-five kilometres with no problem. Hey! It is not worth it. Of course it is not a waste of time, because whether I was sitting, lying or walking – I was thinking about my work. But still, exercise needed to be enhanced by greater effort. I went off to Rost Šport and bought the only poles they

Tomislav Birtić

had that day, Hagan Free Ride Premium. They were telescopic, very, very light, with rubber plugs on the ends. Which, if you are walking on asphalt, and not in nature, you can take off.

What a discovery! I barely covered a kilometre Nordic walking and I had to have a break. But, just as my legs at the beginning of the story could barely cover a kilometre, now it was my arms that were powerless. Everything hurt. My shoulders, upper arms, lower arms. The next day I set off to do a circuit of the lake, but I swung my arms only every other step. I managed to go three quarters of the way around, then I was so tired I had a rest every fifteen minutes and barely completely the circuit.

In my unsuccessful attempts to lose weight I tried several pieces of apparatus I had seen advertised on television. Just like a few of my friends, I bought them, and in the best case scenario they ended up being used as clothes horses, or some of them I gave away. To take up space in someone else's flat. Those walking poles... the best investment in health of all time!

My body adjusted from normal walking to Nordic walking in a week, dramatically more quickly than from no activity to walking. I was excited even after the first miles on the first day. Wonderful! I felt my muscles. Whole muscle groups. My back, shoulders, stomach, chest, even my neck. Under the layers and layers of fat, and years and years of immobility, a real archaeological discovery, a find – muscles.

My legs could last as long as you like. I felt fatigue in my arms, but a month or so later, my arms somehow managed to reach a record, 16,5 miles (26,800 meters) of Nordic walking. Towards the end of the route I felt a pleasant burning sensation in my chest. As though the training was tugging at my muscle fibres like little threads. At the end of the training session, before I had a shower, I went into a café for some coffee and water. I stretched myself happily, and – almost screamed in pain. I had a sharp pain in my stomach muscles. I must have overdone it, it was too great an effort.

"Celebrate, man! Once you were dealing with fat, and now you are talking about muscles," my friend told me.

I had to check whether the pain came from using the poles. The next day, when I started Nordic walking there was no burning in my chest. It came back after five kilometres. As I was walking I folded up the poles, stopped swinging my arms, and the pain immediately disappeared. So, that was it.

For a few days I went crazy because I was not going Nordic walking, because I had been degraded from a sportsman to a normal pedestrian, but this is all normal.

FATE POWERED BY GOOD SHAPE

The manager of the web shop told me to bring the books to the tower block, street and number... And so, I came with a full bag of books in front of the tower, and it was the wrong number. Choosing between the tower and the number, it would have been logical to choose the tower, but I still went another door further on, and chose the number.

"Aaaa, that shop is in the tower block," they told me at the reception desk of the next building.

"Shop? That's on the tenth floor," the receptionist told me, finally, on the ground floor of the tower.

"Web shop? That's on the second floor," the secretary on the tenth floor told me.

"The manager? He's not here. He went out for a meeting." I had no luck on the second floor.

I filled out the delivery form, waited ten minutes, the manager didn't come. So, whatever, I will leave my books, trusting them. We would meet up somehow, so he could sign the forms and bring me the contract.

I went down to the ground floor. It was winter. I moved over to the side not to get in the way of people going in and out of the life, I did up my jacket, pulled my hat down over my ears, and wrapped my scarf around me. And, just to light a cigarette, that was it. Then, a woman, I had never kissed, from my past, from the best prose and poetry, a dream above all dreams. Alive, there, on the spot. Love at first sight, although for us it was the second time.

One of those moments. An almost religious experience. As if God is placing his hands under your feet like steps.

Oh, how glad I was that I had lost 66 pounds (30 kilos). If I hadn't, it would only have been a chance meeting. As it was, weighing 66 pounds less, it was fate. Since, as a charismatic from the Faculty of Philosophy and Social Sciences, professor Despot, said, "Every soul may be everyone's soul," but I add, every body cannot be everyone's body.

Well, that is being in love. I had to deliver the books somewhere else. My hands were shaking. It was the most shaky dedication I had ever written.

"What's up, Tom?" they asked.

"A woman, boys! The Woman!" I replied. "And, the best thing is, it is our destiny. Any resistance is futile. Sometimes life is Babe Ruth. In a trance it shows the way, where it will hit a home run, and the ball actually ends up where it said it would be hit."

"Tom has lost it!" one of them said.

"Off his trolley," another.

"Boys, if this was the reason I had to suffer your comment that you had to air the office for two days after my visit, then today is the day. If I weighed 66 pounds more, I wouldn't have a chance. Nil, zero, nothing, empty set. But now, it is destiny. I look exactly like a thirty-seven year old should look. Six or seven pounds more, on average, precisely so I don't get mobbed by gold diggers and teenagers, but I am attractive to those of twenty-seven to thirty-five, who know what they want and how to get it, whose flats you leave with a smile like an angel."

They rolled about laughing, and I continued drawing hieroglyphics instead of dedications with my trembling hand. I was happy, not for each mile, but for each inch I had walked. I wanted to kiss every inch I had walked.

A few days later she and I had already kissed. Just as I said, it was our destiny. And, as I said, if I hadn't lost 66 pounds...

YOU CAN'T HAVE SEX AS MUCH
AS YOU CAN EAT

I have rarely laughed so loud when reading a newspaper as when I read in 24sata that undoing a bra with one hand burns 22 calories, demanding tantric positions 972 calories, and getting dressed in a hurry with the parents banging on the door, 1218 calories. Sex for twenty minutes a week for a whole year burns as many calories as 75 miles (120 kilometres) of easy jogging. And of course it is clear what people find more pleasant...

True.

However, the five months of the fairy tale of my life, in 2008, also marked the end of the fairy tale of my losing weight. The three best things in the world are the drink before and the cigarette after. Very often we would drink a bottle of red wine at my place. Rarely half each, mainly I would drink two-thirds of the bottle. We would sometimes down quite a lot of brandy, eat a chocolate bar or two. And then the lunches and evening meals. Mainly rich food. Beef steaks, pasta... If she orders meat, I can't eat tomato and mozzarella, and have the entire restaurant laugh at me. And her. The obligatory wine or beer, always a cake, coffee. To put it simply, to repeat the title of this chapter, you really can't have as much sex as you can eat.

In a wink of an eye I had gained 13 pounds (6 kilos), that is I got up to 242 (110), and after we broke up, even more quickly to 253 (115). That relationship, love, was so magnificent, that even the break-up was beautiful, and I did not resort to the typical unisex manoeuvre, drink. But let's say that substituting real values with food did the trick.

OPEN AIR OFFICES AND, YES, THERE IS TIME FOR EXERCISE

"Listen, I think that we shouldn't overburden them by forbidding competition. The damage has already been done, two offices already have our know-how. If we don't let them make a bit on the side, they will be unhappy, and in the end it will come back to haunt us. It is up to you to make sure you get good payback for the favour."

"You know, the main thing in internet advertising now is "click through". Advertisers are paying more attention to what they spend their money on. And until they are convinced that an advertisement is useful where it is, there is no deal. It's a hard fight. They are not interested in how many people saw the ad, but they want concrete evidence that their advertising is beneficial."

"Hm, emphasizing at the meeting that we will get competition sooner or later... Good idea! Yes, and after that only the best will survive, not prosper, but survive."

So, this is what the editor-in-chief of one of the most awarded media in the world, 24sata, said to his three colleagues, as we circled the Sava embankment around the bridges. Here I saw a chance to win the first soul for the light side.

"You see," I told him, "you could have done all this in a stinky office. Or in a café, where you would drink four or five beers. Or even worse, in a restaurant, where you would overeat. And again drink five or six beers."

"I think we know where you are going with this."

"Oh yes. You know. I don't have the time is the excuse. Why don't you come over to join us exercisers?"

He did not become a walker. He chose Pilates. But he came over to the light side. What I want to say is that in many, many cases it is a lie to say you do not have time to exercise. It is not true that you have to be in the office, it is not true that you do not have time to exercise. You cannot sell me that line. Whenever someone tells me they have no time to exercise, I tell him how I used to say that. For years I literally took a paper and pen, and sketched out what my day looked like for well-meaning people, almost triumphantly demonstrating that there were no seconds available for exercise, let alone hours. Then I ended up in the emergency room, then a nervous breakdown, and by some miracle, in those same days, doing the same job, time for walking suddenly appeared.

EL KARNITIN

One of my best friends works for the financial industry. On Friday evenings, his colleagues stagger across the bridge that divides the City from the rest of London. Horrifying stress. For five days investment bankers can control themselves, earning salaries of a hundred thousand or a million pounds and small change a year, and then, on Friday evenings, or Friday night, only one in three or four is capable of walking a straight line. OK, perhaps I am exaggerating, but two hours after the end of the working week they get legless, and become an easy target for binge girls, let alone for the top professional ladies of the night much more suited to their status.

My friend is not at the top of the earning pyramid, but he says that stress is the same on all levels. The struggle for life and death is passionate competition, plus the mortgage crisis and the recession, in which thousands and thousands from the field have become redundant. Although their earnings are more than sufficient to buy healthy food, there is barely time for junk food, and the work is more or less every day, and only the most disciplined amongst them take any exercise. In the time of the worst crisis in their field, he and his friends were not joking when they said that they were working a lot less than before, from seven in the morning until seven at night. They really do work that much. It is presumed that only the lucky ones take less than an hour travelling to work and back. Since my friend enjoys food so much that barbecuing is his favourite hobby – he brings home more pictures of the meat he has cooked from his holidays than a record of his friends – he has had to fight his vice, insisting on living in a flat with a gym in the building.

He revealed to me, and at that time I didn't know how to spell it, "el karnitin". He told me that you could buy it in a pharmacy without a prescription, in tablets or capsules. He recommended the capsules. He convinced me that this substance significantly speeded up weight loss, but there was no point in taking el karnitin if you are not capable of exercising at least an hour and a half without taking a break. You have to take it half an hour before exercise, and it is active for half an hour after you start exercising. In London he does take care of how much he eats, but when he is on holiday he can't resist lamb, sausages, fish... As soon as he gets back to England, in one month he gets back in shape thanks to el karnitin. Of course I had to try it.

L-CARNITINE HELPS EXPRESS WEIGHT LOSS

I went to the pharmacy and asked if they had any el karnitin.

Of course they did. They only had Multipower, but I did not complain.

As my friend suggested, I did not buy the tablets but the liquid, packed in measured tubes. Each tube was three doses.

So, by simply walking at least six miles (ten kilometres) every day, skipping breakfast, eating tomatoes and mozzarella, apple and ham, apple and Emmenthaler cheese, never eating after seven in the evening, I needed to punch another hole in my belt after one month.

Nordic walking and L-Carnitine? I needed a new hole in my belt after a week. If I really let myself go, and went Nordic walking for more often nine than six miles, watching how much, but not so much what and when I ate, allowing myself a sandwich or two, pasta or potatoes, I needed a new hole after two weeks.

"You know, you have to admit in the book that you walked every so often," my financier friend laughed, listening to my enthusiasm about L-Carnitine.

"You think, like you bankers in your contracts, I should admit at least in the small print that it wasn't just a matter of chemicals, that I did have to walk a bit as well?" I laughed with him.

I boasted of the results, obviously losing weight to my friend, my doctor. You look in the mirror and you can't believe your eyes that the fat is melting from your hips and stomach. She told me that I should not take L-Carnitine for longer than three months. But I didn't need any more than that. It burned up the fat much quicker.

Unfortunately, the ease of losing weight, combined with boring walking, was the formula for sudden weight gain. At that time I didn't know what was actually going on, but this is how I flattered myself, not knowing that I was rushing towards serious health problems.

ONLY AGASSI CAN DO THAT, AND ALL OF US WHO ARE FIT

Agassi is the greatest. First he was the greatest talent who had never won anything, nothing major, to win all four. From the perspective of a male pig, Agassi, in the noblest sense of word, is to be envied. He deflowered Brooke Shields (we suppose), married Steffi Graf...

After he had conquered the curse, he beat Ivanišević and won Wimbledon... he did whatever, however he wanted. A little bit of the good life, he put on weight, and then he wanted to get back into perfect shape. And he did. For him the rankings were a walk in the park. Due to the ease of his oscillation between the impression in the uninformed public that his career was coming to an end, and his brilliant performances, he was admired by probably tens of millions of fans. But that is easy.

When I was fat, with a weak ill, several times in a fit of rage against myself I went to the wall. I swore I would hit a ball against the wall until I made a hole in the wall, but I wouldn't last that long. The worst feeling is not being tired, but not having the strength to kill yourself exercising. This is really a bad feeling, to be so unfit that you can't even get truly tired from exercising, because you do not have the strength for more than a few minutes.

My love and I liked the good life. Rich food, slightly lighter booze. But this is the advantage of being man in the best years of life, but fitter than his

Tomislav Birtić

years. The best feeling is to "kill yourself" exercising, but still not be tired. To be so fit, that after one single day the calorimeter tells you that you have burned up four ounces (ten dekagrams) of fat, without that metallic feeling in your chest, and you could exercise for hours more, but you actually aren't tired. Very simply, you feel like a million dollars.

Sometimes I used to think that only a macho man like Agassi could do that. That it was a case of supernatural powers, that you had to be born with it. Today I know that God gave him a forehand, backhand and return that are unforgettable. But, the rest of us are also not so badly off. God gave us, if we are fit, the ability to have to punch two extra holes in our belts as easy as pie. There is nothing better than the freedom of gaining a two or three pounds, when you know you can lose them again at the drop of a hat.

Before the price of ignorance, a little more flattery that leads to problems....

"SON, YOU AND GATTUSSO HAVE THE SAME RESULTS"

"How far does a Champions' League player run?" my old man asked me.

"Let's say that five to six miles (eight or nine kilometres) is enough, everything above ten is very good, and Gattusso probably runs more than seven miles (eleven kilometres)."

"Is that only counting running, or...?"

"No. The computer gives all the data. How much is jogging, how much sprinting, how much walking, and for how many seconds each player stood still on the pitch."

"Super! You walk a little bit more than fore miles (seven kilometres) in an hour, so in an hour and a half, the time a football match lasts, that's six and a half miles (ten and a half kilometres). Fantastic!"

"With extra-time I walk as far as Gattusso runs," I joked.

I was joking, but actually it wasn't a joke.

And neither is this... The first man to swim one thousand five hundred metres in less than fifteen minutes, Vladimir Salnikov, said, "I can give every-one my training plans. The only question is: who can fulfil those plans?" I, however, am giving everyone my training plan, and everyone, I am sure, is capable of fulfilling them and enjoying this similarity with Gattusso.

Tomislav Birtić

The only thing is that I think it would not be good for everyone to follow my weight loss plan, because I am about to write about some serious health issues.

MOUNTAINEERING,
BURNING FAT IN REAL TIME

My friend was a mountain climber. Nothing spectacular, nothing dangerous, no ropes, no alpinism, just delightful walking uphill and downhill, in nature.

For years he tried to persuade me, and finally, when walking and even Nordic walking were no longer any real effort, I agreed to go up a mountain, Sljeme, with him and his friends. In contrast to walking on the flat, where I would very simply reach the maximum speed you can attain when walking, let's say about five miles (eight kilometres) an hour, and I could maintain that easily without my pulse changing at all, climbing was a revelation. I immediately got out of breath. Although the first part of the climb was very easy, I could not talk while I was walking. That gentle climb was a huge, huge effort for me. But just as I did when I started walking on flat ground, I would stop. Plus, I enjoyed the beautiful scenery, and drank spring water. The air was also a revelation. We city dwellers actually have no idea what clear air is. Fresh and clean. I enjoyed it, I breathed deeply. Halfway up the six hundred metre climb, we took a break, and then followed a horribly difficult climb for me, up to the mountain hut. I had to stop every fifteen minutes. Although I hardly made it, and considered giving up at least ten times, still, sensing that beautiful metal taste of effort in my lungs for the first time since my teenage years, I climbed to the top, ate the

Tomislav Birtić

best bean stew with sausages, and drank the sweetest beer in my life. It was all new to me, and I was surprised to find that going down the mountain was just as tiring. It was easier, but it was also tiring. When you climb you strain your motor, but when you are coming down you use your suspension and brakes.

The most important thing for my good will was that at the foot of the climb I had tightened my belt, and when we got to the mountain hut I was able to tighten it half a hole, but not yet an entire hole.

OVEREATING AND 1 POUND
(HALF A KILO) LESS

So here we are in May 2009. There was no way I could get below 253 pounds (115 kilos). Fortunately I spent more of the time slightly above 253 than slightly below 264 (120 kilos).

Location: Bjelolasica, photo safari with Stjepan. The one who complimented me on not smelling.

On Friday night I drank five beers. While waiting for dinner I ate a lot of bread. And then, the starter: carbonnara, main course: veal with roast potatoes, mixed salad, and two custard pies. Of course, two beers after dinner.

Saturday breakfast: two fried eggs, then last of all the remains of an omelette, three frankfurters, and corn flakes with milk.

Three hours hiking through the wood, that is, the photo safari. For a man who was meeting with rocks for the first time, the going was pretty unpleasant. I used up quite a lot of energy just keeping my balance.

Before lunch: two beers and a Schwepps, and then a large steak with an egg and vegetables, with beer of course, two cakes with cheese and nuts.

And then two more hours photo safari.

Before dinner a beer, and for dinner: soup, two large pieces of chicken with roast potatoes, salad, and a cake with nuts and chocolate. I ate so much that Stjepan felt ill just watching me gobble it all down.

Tomislav Birtić

Breakfast: a full plate of omelette and frankfurters, and corn flakes, and then we went home.

As soon as I got into my flat and stood on the scales I had a shock. One pound (half a kilo) less than before Bjelolasica!

"Altitude," my friend said, hearing about my report from the photo hike.

"No idea... I didn't want to be a wet blanket so I ate and drank like crazy. I was prepared for increased effort when I got back, to stop stuffing my face, and would you believe, I weighed 1 pound less. I really don't know what to think. Hiking through the woods, due to the terrain, I had to keep my balance all the time. Because of the rocks and branches, all kinds of obstacles, you have to be careful you don't fall all the time, and you are holding a camera in your hands and a rucksack on your back. And it did occur to me that it had something to do with altitude."

"What do you think, why do so many teams go to the mountains to prepare for a match?"

"It looks like that is the reason. What would I have looked like if I had eaten that lot at home?! Like I am careful what I eat? It seems I lost 10 pounds just like that. No more summer holidays on the coast. Mountains, mountains and nothing but mountains – that is, hills."

I sent a message to my doctor, Željko Šućur. "I was on Bjelolasica on a photo safari, which is actually three plus two hours hiking. From Friday evening to Sunday morning I ate so much it was frightening, the worst possible combinations, and washed it all down with at least ten beers. I lost 1 pound. Is that because of the altitude?"

"It is important that you have clearly become really fit, so your metabolism automatically speeds up," he replied.

Yes... This is a good moment to mention that all men in all countries know everything about football, and all women and all men in all countries know all about losing weight and everything to do with losing weight. I was on Bjelolasica just two days, and I imagined that I, although I ate like crazy, had lost weight due to the altitude. The altitude in the basin where we were walking was 620 m. What a wise guy!

It is also a good moment to mention again that I should have talked to a doctor ages and ages ago. Or several of them. When I got back from Bjelolasica I immediately called a friend and arranged to climb Učka on the following weekend. Because, Sljeme, a kilometre closer to the Sun, was not enough, I was going for greater heights. Seven months later I was almost a cripple. But we will get around to that...

"DO YOU SEPARATE THE FAT OFF YOUR HAM?" THE ZONE DIET

After a circuit round the lake I came across the world swimming record holder, world runner-up and European champion Gordan Kožulj. We had met before because as a journalist I had written about him. This is one of those happy acquaintances that borders on friendship. Happy because after the last round of the World Cup, in Paris, he was permitted to live in a slightly unsporting manner, and I spent several unforgettable hours with the Kožulj family. With some people you just "click," it is not "journalist-sportsman," but man to man.

"What are you doing here?" he asked, after we had said hello.

"Well, I have done a circuit round Jarun. I am losing weight."

"Well done! How are you losing weight?"

"I walk at least six miles (ten kilometres) every day..."

"Great!" he interrupted me. "Walking is the healthiest exercise."

"And I also watch what I eat," I completed my description of my method.

"What are you going to eat this evening?"

"Apple and ham."

"Do you separate the fat off your ham?"

"Hey, Gordan, I am not training to break the world record!" I laughed, "I only want to reach my ideal weight, or at least to get as close to it as possible.

I don't have breakfast. I eat either tomato and mozzarella or apple and ham."

"How much have you lost so far?"

"Sixty six pounds. (Thirty kilos.)"

"What!? Sixty six pounds! In how much time?"

"In a little over four months, five months... Well, to be honest, first I lost 66 pounds, but recently I have gained a bit over 22 pounds (10 kilos).

"We haven't seen each other for a long time, let's have a drink." He immediately said he had never had any problems losing weight, but it was hard to put on weight and maintain his weight, so perhaps he was not the best person to talk on this subject.

"So I don't have any kind of experience with losing weight, but I think that physical activity is best for that. The most unhealthy thing a person can do if he wants to lose weight is just reduce what he eats. Your body needs food. See, I am at the end of my career, but I am still training because my body feels better after physical activity. Effort produces endorphins, and other hormones that make you happy..." said Gordan.

"What should a recreational sportsman eat who has decided to lose weight?"

"What you have just said is actually not bad at all. Except it is a mistake not to eat breakfast, and what you are eating is monotonous. I used to stick to the "The Zone Diet", the book written by Dr. Barry Sears. The book was very popular in America while I was studying there. "The Zone Diet" talks about a balanced diet, in a ratio of 40-30-30, in terms of carbohydrates, proteins and fats. The ratios are not about quantity but energy value. I went to a few of his lectures. Sears talked about how a professional

Tomislav Birtić

sportsman's diet is not very different from the diets of ordinary people. Sportsmen are too focused on carbohydrates as the main source of energy. In everyday life fats play an important role. But, of course, you have to know how to differentiate between fats, not all fats are the same. Saturated, unsaturated, animal, plant origin. I ate as he said, and above all I was healthier. My problem was that I got over-tired during training sessions. My immunity fell, and I got sick. Sears talked about how food is not just food, but also medicine. But, for a recreational sportsman to lose weight, he has to have a balanced diet. One of the most important foods "in the zone" is Mediterranean food, because everything you mentioned is there. Vegetables – tomatoes – are very important. Mozzarella is exceptional! There is also fish, and ham has its place, if you watch the quantity, and especially if you take the fatty part off the red meat. Apple and ham? Excellent! Ham is also good with melon. So, what you were doing is great. Fruit, vegetables, protein – a super combination. Only, since you were on a strict diet, you should take vitamins and minerals in tablet form."

"Why?"

"If you eat monotonous food for a long time, however good it is, your body will be lacking some important elements. That is why it is necessary to take dietary supplements. If you don't eat enough fish, you should take omega 3 fatty acids. There is also omega 6 and omega 9, but omega 3 is the main one. They are important for brain function and your blood system. Before they used to say, "Don't eat that, it's fatty," but those fatty acids, taken after a heart attack, reduce deaths by forty per cent. So, if you don't eat fish and nuts, or don't use linseed oil, you need to take omega acids. If you are losing weight, you must reduce your meals. However much you exercise, while you are losing weight, you also need to eat less. That's why you need to take vitamins and minerals in tablet form."

"But... I didn't mix proteins and carbohydrates, and in my fanatical phase I only ate fruit after six in the evening. The richest thing I ate after six was a banana, but mainly only apples. Or salad. Plus walking at least six miles (ten kilometres) a day. Like that, I needed a new hole in my belt in a month. About 13 pounds (6 kilos) a month. What should I have eaten?"

"There are some serious scientists who say that you shouldn't eat proteins and carbohydrates together. But I am not a fan of that diet. Everything plays a role. For proteins to be absorbed better, it is necessary to eat carbohydrates after them, because they raise your insulin, and help the nutrients to be "pushed" to your cells. Also, if you are a recreational sportsman and you want to lose weight, you shouldn't eat anything at all after eight, or at least nothing serious. You said you didn't eat after six, but that is too extreme. You could have eaten fish. I really love sea fish especially. But any fish is great for you. And you were wrong not to eat breakfast. Breakfast is really the most important meal, because it gives you energy for the whole day."

"Is that really true?"

"That is really true."

And then he dictated an eating plan for me.

Tomislav Birtić

THE EATING PLAN OF THE WORLD RECORD HOLDER FOR THE 100 M AND 200 M BACKSTROKE

"What do you have for breakfast?" I asked, him, that is the world vice-champion, the winner of the World Cup, the European champion, Gordan Kožulj.

"Oat flakes."

"With milk?"

"You can eat them with milk."

"Yes, but what do you eat them with?"

"Some people eat them with orange juice, so they at least taste of something. But that juice also has calories."

"OK, what do you eat oat flakes with?"

"With water. If you take something with a lot of calories during the day, then oat flakes are the best choice for breakfast. Corn flakes are also alright, or muesli. You can, to get some protein, have an egg too, but only the white. Sometimes I used to eat Čokolino (children's cereal with oats and chocolate) regularly in the mornings. I tried to eat five to six meals a day. Since I had to train at 7 in the morning I had breakfast at 6.30. After the morning session, I would have a protein shake at 9.30. Then I would have breakfast again, about 10.30, my second breakfast, but third meal. Lunch was at 1 in the afternoon."

"What was for lunch?"

"Fish, turkey, chicken or veal. Along those lines it is possible to create a menu for recreational sportsmen too. The only thing is that for recreational sportsmen it is enough to eat one turkey breast, in olive oil."

"What would you combine the meat with? Did you eat it with potatoes or just with salad?"

"Well, I ate meat with potatoes, but I wouldn't recommend that for other people. My recommendation for recreational sportsmen would be meat, in olive oil, seasoned to taste, and salad."

"And then?"

"My second training session began at 4 p.m. Halfway through the training I would drink a protein shake, and I would have supper quite late, because I wouldn't get home until 9."

"And supper was?"

"For me it was full of calories. I had something similar for supper as I had had for lunch. Plus, I would boost my supper with protein, because we grow while we are resting. Training is stress. It is a series of micro-traumas, bursting fibres. During training you lose weight, that is, you get smaller. You only grow if your body rests."

Aha! This world record holder has opened up a whole new chapter!

CATABOLISM, OR: WHY SLEEP IS IMPORTANT AND WHAT PROTEINS FOR SUPPER ARE FOR

"Why did I, suffering from insomnia, lose weight in a bad way?" I continued to ask the great expert in nutrition, and each minute it was clearer. I don't know what Nobel Prize winners might have said, but Gordan was great. "I was happy with the pace I lost weight only at times when I was sleeping well," I said.

"Children who do not sleep well tend to get fatter more. Sportsmen, if they want to put on weight before a competition, have to eat a lot of protein before bed. A sportsman has to take amino acids. There is a phase during sleep called catabolism. We usually sleep eight hours. Just before the end of our sleep, our body usually begins to eat itself, because we have not eaten anything for eight hours. So, in order for your body to have energy for your heart, brain etc. to function, it eats itself. In order to maintain our weight, we sportsmen have to eat more protein before sleeping. Not carbohydrates, because they contain insulin, and it causes a hormone to increase that is produced during stress, cortisol, which goes on to cause catabolism. Therefore, I would eat eggs or meat before going to bed, or pure whey, or amino acids in liquid form. From the fifth to the eighth hour of sleep the body goes into catabolism. That means, your body has used up the food it received before sleep, and begins to eat its reserves. If you don't have any reserves of fat, your body eats its own muscles. Sleep is important. For those who want to lose weight, sleep is also an opportunity. But I would recommend that they also eat proteins rather than carbohydrates. If you sleep well, you will lose weight more easily. The last two to three hours of sleep are pure weight loss."

"So that is it... You, as a top sportsman, have to make sure your organism doesn't eat itself. But for me as a recreational sportsman that is great. I have a nice snooze and my organism eats up my fat."

"That's right. The only thing is, don't eat carbo-hydrates before bed, and try not to eat after eight o'clock. The time from eight in the evening until (depending on when you get up) seven, eight or nine in the morning, is important for losing weight. Your body eats itself."

"The last few days, purely by chance, some people have told me the fairy tale of L-Carinitine. Is that a fairy tale? Or does it really help?"

"L-Carnitine is old. It speeds up your metabolism, that is, it speeds up use of fat."

"So it is true? It is not just a marketing trick by the pharmaceutical industry?"

"L-Carnitine is a regular ingredient of dietary nu-trition for losing weight. They say it helps you burn fat more easily. It is used for sport and recreation."

Tomislav Birtić

THE RECOMMENDATION OF A WORLD RECORD HOLDER: IF I WANT TO LOSE FAT, I HAVE TO GO TO THE GYM, AND CROSSOVER

"You have not had problems with excess weight. But how have your colleagues dealt with that problem?" I brought him back to the subject that interested me most.

"Many people don't know and many neglect the fact that the gym will be much more useful than aerobic training like walking. In the research I have read, it has been shown that, if you work out in the gym, your accelerated metabolism lasts longer than when you do aerobic training. Your metabolism, for accelerated burning of fat cells, if you walk actively, quickly for an hour or two, is only active while you are walking. If you go to the gym, or do something more strenuous, your metabolism is accelerated for those two hours in the gym, plus two hours after you have exercised. I suppose this is because your body has become used to walking through evolution. It is very efficient when you walk. On the other hand, the gym causes your muscles greater stress. Our bodies have not evolved to be used to heavy weight. So our metabolism takes longer to break through that situation, that stress."

"Fantastic!"

"However thin they are, marathon runners have a higher percentage of fat in their subcutaneous tissue than body builders. It has been shown that this is because, after you have worked out in the gym, your metabolism continues to work for hours after training. When you run, walk or swim... your organism returns to its normal position more quickly. What happens? First you use adenosine triphosphate (ATP). That gets going as soon as you do. After a minute. In the next ten minutes you get rid of glycogen and then you move on to your fat reserves. You train your body to use fat as a source of energy if you walk for two hours every day, or run for an hour, or swim for two hours. Your body gets used to using your fat as a source of energy. But, when you eat, your body stores the fat better."

"Stores it?! Like I'm going to need it?!"

"Precisely. A lot of long-haul sportsmen, regardless of which sport they are in, have an awful lot of fat. So, under stress your body says: "Uh! I need this, I will store it! And you start going round in circles. In order to burn fat, instead of two hours you have to walk for three. The human body is incredibly clever. Incredibly adaptable. Your body thinks: "What do I need to do to survive? A-ha! That's it!" And it is very intelligent, it does it really well. Whatever activity you are involved in, your body reasons: "I have experienced stress. I will try to go back to how it was, just in case, I will create reserves, and I will try not to come under that kind of stress again". That is how you get muscles. In the gym you work hard, your fibres snap, in a series of micro-traumas, your body falls. You give it time to rest, your body returns to where it was, and by so-called supercompensation, it builds muscles."

"Your body is actually defending itself from us?"

Tomislav Birtić

"That's right; your body is defending itself. It is telling you: "You have caused me terrible stress. I don't want to be in that situation, ever, and certainly never again!"

"What was my body saying? In four months of asceticism I lost 66 pounds (30 kilos), looked great. And then I started living the dolce vita with my love. Dinners, lunches, less exercise... You are in fact telling me that my organism could hardly wait for me to end my asceticism, so my body immediately, very quickly accumulated reserves? That means, whoever starts physical activity is condemned to continue with it forever? As soon as you stop, you're done for?"

"There is room for manipulation. After your body learns to use certain energy for survival, as soon as you use that up, your body will replace it most quickly. You have got your body used to long walks, for which your body uses fat. Your body will sooner store fat in the old places than mine, because my activity is different."

"As soon as it gets the chance, my body will store energy in that store place?"

"In the form of fat!"

"So, that is those steaks with gnocchi, that my love and I ate? My body said: "Yes! I am putting this away!"?"

"Yes. And now it won't store its energy in glycogens or ATP, but as quickly as possible in fat. So, long distance runners have a higher percentage of fat than body builders, because their bodies need more fat. The body will say: "I have been using that most for five years now," and of course it will store it there the quickest."

"So, the ideal form of exercise would be...?"

"The trend in the world nowadays is some form of crossover, half an hour running or walking and half an hour in the gym. That is optimal. After training like that your body won't need to put back everything you eat as fatty tissue, but it will store it in other energy zones."

"Why is walking the healthiest form of exercise?"

"Because it is the most natural for us."

"Because man was made to walk?"

"Precisely. We have evolved like that."

"I chose walking because I weighed 295 pounds (134 kilos) and I was in terrible shape. Running would have killed my ankles..."

"Precisely. Swimming is good too, because you move without any burden on your joints. But if you don't know how to swim and breathe properly you will get tired too quickly. Many people say: "I am going swimming to lose some weight". But, in order to succeed, you have to be able to swim for long enough. To burn the fat, you have to swim long enough. People start, but they don't know how to breathe properly, and because they don't breathe correctly they lose their breath too quickly and stop. They are not physically tired, but they stop."

"So, what is breathing properly?"

"To breathe in and fill your lungs and breathe out. People usually breathe too shallow."

"Give us recreational sportsmen some recommendations. Let's say, I am going on holiday, I want to swim, what is best for me?"

"It is best to do the breast stroke. Then your head is always above the water, it is the easiest. Correct breathing, in all aerobic activities, helps you to lose weight. It's a simple law of physics: oxygen helps

Tomislav Birtić

burning. Walking is more natural, most people find it easier to lose weight by walking. Running is too much for a lot of people, too much effort. Also, water is colder than air, so your metabolism works more slowly. Walking is also better for losing weight because, due to the air temperature, because of the sun, it raises the body to a higher temperature, so the metabolism works faster. In swimming all your muscles are at work, which is not the case with walking."

"But that is why we have Nordic walking. All your muscles are at work, except your facial muscles."

"Precisely. A robot working with its feet alone uses batteries more slowly than a robot that works with its hands and feet. It is the same with people. We also have energy batteries."

If I had only listened to him. The world record holder, the sportsman, a man who reads the latest research every day, told me what to do, what to eat, but I continued to do it my way. The price was terrible.

AFTER A RECORD AND LUNCH
I SAW STARS

That day the weather was ideal for mountain walking. Neither hot nor cold, just nice. A dry path, and soft.

I had coffee with my friend, who drove me to the bottom of the path, and set off. I climbed more easily than before. Incredibly easily. As if I were a balloon, and not made of flesh and blood. And bones. Often I would drink half a litre of water before the first break. This time I didn't drink a drop, I didn't even get breathless. Usually the break at the resting place half way up was very welcome. I would sit on the bench for about ten minutes, talk with other hikers I met there, or just enjoy listening to the birds or the wind, and then I would carry on. This time I stopped, just for the sake of prevention. I thought, it is impossible, just like that, all at once, so suddenly in comparison with the previous time, to walk uphill like I could on level ground. Afraid that my body was suffering from strain, which I could not feel in my excitement, I sat on the bench for literally three minutes and drank two or three mouth fulls of water.

I climbed up to the last and steepest part of the path just as easily, wondering just as much how I was taking that part of the path all of a sudden without any effort, almost without losing breath. I had to slow down by sheer force of will, because I was climbing not just easily, but also very quickly, of course in relation to my previous times. I slowed down and en-

Tomislav Birtić

joyed the scenery. I was very proud of myself. From a fatty who had to stop every few hundred metres when walking, I had advanced to mountain climbing with ease. I felt as though I could carry on climbing until the day after tomorrow.

The craziest thing was that I felt like this at the steepest part. I climbed without a pause, I wasn't even thirsty. The only thing was I felt something low down in my back. It wasn't a pain, just a feeling. I arrived at the mountain hut somehow too early. I was almost disappointed that the climb was over (from mountain hut to the top is not a climb, more a walk). I was enjoying myself so much I didn't want to join the crowd on the terrace or in the restaurant just yet. For a moment I sat down on a tree stump by the hut. The stump was cold, so I stood up and stood for five minutes, listening to the wind.

It was all by the book. I got dry and changed my clothes in the hut. That day the beans and sausage were better than usual. And the white cabbage was even better. And so it was, until I tried to get up from the table. I felt an intense pain in my back. I didn't scream, but I groaned so loud that the entire room heard me. Like in a cartoon, and who knew that it is no joke but true to life, I saw stars it hurt me so much.

I walked up to the top, then got a bus down to the tram terminal. I barely made it out of the bus, and I barely managed to limp to the tram and then home. Of course, the real pain began after I had cooled down. And this brings us slowly to the small print in many books, or to the part of the television commercial where the voice-over reads the text as quickly as possible but still being comprehensible. Ask your doctor. Before you do it, ask your doctor. Publishers and writers write this to avoid court cases. Some write it so it is barely legible, in tiny letters, tiny like those in a contract where the other party is to be stripped naked. Others are, I suppose, so afraid of being sued, that they don't play about with small print, but they actually emphasize the warning. I will put the warning on the cover, not for legal reasons, but because I have experienced in my own flesh, the reason for that exalted advice. How much time I would have saved, it would not have hurt, how much more I would have enjoyed being in the countryside (and various groups of friends) and I could have lost weight so much more quickly, if I had listened to the advice to ask my doctor, to talk to a doctor. The good thing was, the person I did not go to for advice, for tests, although he had been offering them to me for years, so I had to go to see him now for safe therapy, had treated no less than the winner of the skiing World Cup, the world champion, the winner of a silver Olympic medal, Ivica Kostelić, and the best handball player of all time, Ivano Balić etc. etc. ...

Dr. Slobodan Kuvalja and I are even friends. I had interviewed him, and after the interview we chatted about all kinds of things. We became friends. But, if I hadn't known anything about him except that he had made Kostelić fit and ready to make history, that would have been enough for me to go straight to him. And I also knew that Cybex was developed by NASA, so astronauts could exercise in a state of weightlessness, and about the experience of my friends who had come away from Kuvalja as though re-born...

I called him. I described what my happy day with the unhappy ending had looked like. He asked if my

Tomislav Birtić

legs were numb, I said my right leg was numb to my knee, and, to cut a long story short, he told me to lie down until it got better. If it should hurt, I should take some Brufen immediately. He strictly forbade me to climb even after the pain passed, and this time he simply ordered me to come to the Cybex centre for an examination.

KUVALJA USED CYBEX TO GET KOSTELIĆ AND BALIĆ READY TO MAKE HISTORY, AND ME TO EXERCISE FOR FUN

To overcome my embarrassment, my fear of tests, which might show what I do not want to hear, I asked Kuvalja why I had had that pain in my back. OK, I am a recreational sportsman, but it didn't hurt me like that when I could hardly make the climb, but precisely on that outing when I felt like I was flying up the mountain. So... If you cool a muscle, especially if it is having problems, weak, irritated, in spasm, the muscle will contract. I was walking in the winter, I sat on a stump. Just enough to bare my back. Why do we cool injuries? For instance, if you hit a muscle, so the blood vessels contract, so there is no large bruise, and to calm the painful reaction. However, what is important in my case, the muscle, when it gets very cold, shrivels up. It gets shorter. If the muscles are not equally strong, then they will shrink unevenly, and as they do so they will shift parts of the construction. That is why I had that pain in my back. Unequally strong muscles shifted the structure, which pressed on my nerves, and I suffered pain. Most often it gets you in the summer. You sweat, and the wind blows gently over the sweaty part of your body. Most often it is in your neck and back, the most sensitive parts, where the neural structures, the nerves, are close by. That is when physics kicks in. Evaporation of liquid is increased. For liquid to evaporate it takes energy. As a result there is a fall in temperature on the base,

Tomislav Birtić

in this case your skin. It is transferred downwards, deep inside to your muscles. Your muscle goes into spasm. It compresses, shrivels. Farmers know a trick about cooling water melons. They cover the water melon with a wet cloth. The water evaporates from the cloth, and the water melon is colder than the air around it.

My condition... I was struck by pain in my right hip. When I was sitting and especially when I was walking. My right knee was not so good either. I avoided putting any weight on it. Kuvalja asked me about my job, my way of life, my activities, exercise, and I told him. I told him I work sitting down. I had been eating take-away lunches, mainly meat and potatoes. I was inactive, and I put on a huge amount of weight. Due to a combination of stress, age and years of poor diet and no exercise, I had pains in my chest. I ended up in the emergency room. The doctor told me that if I didn't do something with myself, for myself, I could die. I decided to lose weight, but I was losing weight without professional help. I starved myself, and I walked at least six miles (ten kilometres) every day. For months I walked home from work, and I ate only light, over light lunches, and even lighter suppers. First I lost the water from my body, then some fat, and in the end I was using up my muscles. With the remainders of my muscles, since walking on flat ground after several months was no longer tiring, I began climbing Sljeme, and other hills. Right up until I got that pain in my back.

And so I came to the Cybex centre, almost disabled. Kuvalja weighed me. He asked me how tall I was. He put all this information, and my sex, into his computer and then tested the dodgy parts of my body.

The tests showed that some of my muscles were lacking up to sixty per cent of their strength. Unexpectedly poor results for my age, weight and the rest. But the tests corresponded with the problems that had made me contact him: back pain, numbness in my legs, a hunched spine. And, yes, I was a typical patient who had suffered a variety of diets, with inexpert weight loss causing a great deal of fat to be melted, but also muscle mass, and as a result I had become very weak.

"You were so weak, that we didn't know if the therapy would work on you," Kuvalja told me later. "When a patient comes to us as standard post-operative procedure, with such weak, loose muscles, in that phase we first of all have to work with electricity, and only after that with isokinetics. But, since you were not injured, there was no trauma, we started Cybex immediately on you, which proved to be a good choice."

After only two sessions of exercise, the pain in my hip disappeared, and after only five days, I cleaned my shower, crouching down for several minutes, which I had not been able to do for years. Or, my hobby is photography, and with absolutely no trouble I took several pictures, which had been inaccessible to me for years because I was unable to crouch and keep still, or kneel on one knee. Why is Cybex so effective?

"When I do analyses, ergonomics are extremely important, and life style and work going back five, six or ten years," says Kuvalja. "I always ask my patients that. Ten years ago you were sitting, smoking, drinking beer after beer, and eating bad food. You put on weight and you did no exercise. You increased the

Tomislav Birtić

weight on your structure, and the structure lost the ability to carry that weight. As if the tyres on your car were always losing air a little, but you kept on loading more and more weight into the car, and in the end they got down to the wheel rims. On the other hand, you did not have any serious injuries at all, or operations, or illnesses that affected your joints and muscles. The pain you felt in your back is the result of disturbed statics and bio-mechanics. You overdid it. In isokinetics the involvement of the muscles is completely adjusted to the physiology of the muscle fibres. When the muscle fibres get shorter, and when they relax, they are of a certain length, they pull certain parts in the joint and thereby develop a certain level of force. That force is different for every angle of movement of the joint, depending on the length of the muscle fibre. In isokinetics, which is why these systems were invented, the machine communicates with the joint muscles. It communicates at least at every 0.4 degrees of movement. Let's take a knee. The axis of the knee joint and the axis of the dynamometer are synchronized. The muscle moves, and the burden on the joint is negligible. The burden is on the muscle. That is why a patient with a badly damaged knee has pain in his knee when he walks. The damaged cartilage hurts, but while he is working on an isokinetics machine it does not hurt, because the joint is moved to the side and the burden is on the muscle. On that principle, the muscle is under the optimal burden in every position, from maximum to minimum extension. The electricity tones the muscle. It can strengthen it, to make it firmer, but it cannot teach it in which position it needs to place the joint. This comes from an order by the brain, related to position, gravity, weight and the desire for movement. Isokinetic rehabilitation is called neuromuscular rehabilitation, because the patient moves according to orders from the brain. When we are using electricity, that has nothing to do with the brain. Here we are working on the entire chain: the brain, the nerves that produce signals, the muscle, the receptors, the joint. Second, your muscles were healthy, they were just neglected. You were like a parked car. A car on its wheel rims. You think that someone punctured your tyres. However, no one slashed them, but there is no air in the tyres. You blow up the tyres, balance them, you get in, start the car and drive off. And what is very important, your tyres were not inflated evenly. When you start doing isokinetics, since the fibres are involved the entire time, your muscles get their strength back five or even eight times faster than in the gym. You do isotonic movements with weights, which means the muscle always has the same resistance. We said that the muscle stretches and shortens depending on the angle of the joint, and at every angle it needs a different force, a different level of resistance. This means that with your knee bent at ninety degrees, when you want to stretch it out, you need a certain number of Newtons, for the next few degrees another number of Newtons, and so on. And vice versa. Secondly, you have to do it synchronized, in both directions. People's movement are synchronized. Both legs have to work. An isokinetics machine communicates with the patient and at every moment provides the level of resistance he needs, in order to make progress. No more, no less. That is why you have made such quick progress. As soon as we had worked a few days with you, and you

Tomislav Birtić

had healthy muscles, just empty, you were able to increase the strength of your empty muscles by up to twenty per cent a day. In a few days we managed to return a lot of strength, and your body recognized that immediately. The parts stopped moving, and they no longer hurt."

The procedure was so successful, that I, as I said, previously almost disabled, left Cybex like a sportsman. The problems of my hips, knee and spine were resolved. After the therapy I could walk up to the fifteenth floor, without stopping of course, and my pulse rose by five beats. (There was a crowd waiting for the lift. My neighbour was taking up some furniture, and suddenly there were as many people on the ground floor as at a tram stop at seven a.m. I couldn't be bothered to wait my turn, so I started to climb. At a regular fast pace, I walked up, as though I was walking on flat ground. I did not slow down, let alone take a break. Although I was wearing a T-shirt, a shirt, jumper and jacket, I did not sweat a drop. And my pulse increased by only five beats. Truly rehabilitated. A sportsman). I climbed Sljeme, in places trampling through snow up to my knees, without a break. Kuvalja told me that I had a healthy cardiovascular system, which reacted to training by becoming fit. By exercising the muscles in my knees, hips and spine, I was also exercising my heart muscle and my blood vessels. If we neglect our muscles, the small blood vessels, capillaries, do not supply sufficient blood, that is they supply as much as the muscles need for that small amount of movement. A weak person starts to run, but insufficient blood gets through the capillaries, the muscle is suffocated and his legs hurt. He can't do it. His heart isn't necessarily pounding.

He just can't. When a healthy person starts exercising, with isokinetics he is also exercising his heart muscle. In countries that are rich enough, these exercises are used for heart patients, because the effort is optimized. You can't do the patient any harm. If he is finding it hard, he stops. In contrast to running on a treadmill, which does not stop, so the patient could even die. This means, when you are exercising like that, your heart muscle is exercised to cover the needs of the organs, in this case, the muscles. Secondly, if necessary, it encourages an increase in the number of capillaries on the peripheries, which supply the muscles with blood, to improve the supply of oxygen to that tissue.

From then on, I have been going to Cybex twice a year, and every eighteen months for a complete test. I am a mountain climber. I climb, and the muscles in my backside become stronger. The muscles which pull my knees up to my chin have nothing to do. And so misbalance occurs. This will displace the position of the hips, meaning that the pelvis is twisted, and in the end the spine will have problems.

"In my experience," says Kuvalja, "Cybex works for several years before the problem returns. A patient with a guitar band asked me why he had to be tested again. Hadn't he solved his problem? I asked him what is the first thing he does when he goes to play in a bar. He tunes his strings. I asked him why he tunes them if he tuned them yesterday. They have gone out of tune, there is no harmony. There is a percentage of tolerance which does not cause problems, ten per cent is not a problem. But, after you go too far, the construction is shaken, until it finally collapses. In my experience, a year and a half is the time in which

Tomislav Birtić

the muscles do not have time to get out of tune so much to cause damage. They can last for even four or five years. I remember a patient who came back after fourteen years – for a "service". That old lady is eighty-four years old. But... In younger people, as they are working, the time is shorter. Stress takes a terrible toll."

Kuvalja rehabilitated a mutual friend. She left Cybex for the coast as a sportswoman. She swam for miles with no trouble. Running, wonderful. Not long after she came back from her holiday she went back to Cybex, out of sorts just as she was the first time she went there. As though they hadn't done anything. Stress. A year and a half to two is the ideal time for a precise check-up. There is no new damage, you are in top form the whole time, you are protected from injuries and the least possible exercise is needed to get back in top shape.

And after he had not only rehabilitated me, but made me into a sportsman, Kuvalja recommended to me....

MASAI BAREFOOT TECHNOLOGY, ANTI-SHOES

The Swiss anti-shoe manufacturer, Masai Barefoot Technology (MBT) heard that Kuvalja was using isokinetics. They came for an interview, and asked him what he thought of their technology. He studied MBT, and understood what it is.

What is it all about? The Masai have no problems with their loco-motor system. That is well-known. Scientists studied why. First, biomechanical analysis. They studied ergonomics, and concluded that the Masai walk as upright as a candle. If you watch them on television, you can see they are straight. None of them have hunched shoulders. Apart from sick people. Then they noticed that they walk barefoot. And the ground they walk on is sandy. As a result the Masai have differently configured heels. When a Masai takes a step, his heel sinks deep into the sand. And then the whole foot goes further. Scientists realized that the point is that they have to move forward from where their heel has sunk into the sand. Then they went to make shoes with a substance in the sole that would imitate that movement. On MBT shoes, there is a special red substance in the back, which sinks down when you stand on it. And then you step forward. Successful simulation.

"Excellent for prevention, good for maintenance of your condition after rehabilitation, but not good for treatment. First you have to reset the system. Those shoes are not made to strengthen an isolated

Tomislav Birtić

group of muscles separately. Someone who has a damaged meniscus, meaning one of his muscles is weaker, and it is shaky as a result, could have more problems from those shoes. If someone has problems with their knees or hips, wearing MBT could make it worse," Kuvalja told me. "Until it is reset. But after you reset it, they are good for maintenance. Or for prevention, which is what they were created for."

I bought MBT shoes because Kuvalja recommended them. It's simple. I came to see him, almost disabled, I left him like a sportsman, so of course I will do what he says, although anti-shores are quite expensive, between 200 and 250 dollars. It is true, they last for years, but they are expensive.

Silly me. He told me not to walk in anti-shoes at first for more than fifteen minutes. The first day I walked about six miles (ten kilometres). My arms hurt, but not my legs. Why my arms?

"You had pain from your back and shoulders," Kuvalja explained to me. "Because the shoes changed your position. They made you walk upright. The muscles which had not yet been exercised, in the neck and back, got tired. So they complained. But your legs have already been broken in, so they stood the effort better."

And, Dr. Kuvalja recommended something else to me.

NINTENDO WII FIT, LOSING WEIGHT WAS NEVER THIS MUCH FUN

Kuvalja's patient came for a check-up after quite a long time. The tests were much better than otherwise after a long break. He asked her if there was anything new in her life style. She replied: "Well I bought a Nintendo, and I exercise all the time." He went on the internet. He saw that it was some form of simulation. He studied all the available material, watched the exercises, and decided that that was it.

"The Japanese have realized that it is really important. One of those people, like me, was their advisor, but they, to sell more, made it like a game," he said. "But it is exercise. Made very cleverly. It's great. Very useful in old people's homes. You can't give old people so much strength back. But! In the joints, tendons, the brain, you have receptors which show you where you are. People have perfect sensors. However, if they get rusty, if you don't exercise, you become clumsy. Older people, if they exercise using a Nintendo, become more dexterous, better protected, more capable. But it is in fact a toy. Nintendo is a very useful toy."

I loved the game from the film First Knight. When Richard Gere overcomes obstacles to win the right to kiss Julia Ormond. The first time I exercised I made a puddle of sweat one metre wide around the base. I love the balance and step exercises. I bought the EA Sport Active Personal Trainer, and then the Active Personal Trainer 2, because there is a gadget in

Tomislav Birtić

it that measures your pulse. Mostly I boxed, great cardio exercise, and there are also exercises with a stretch band...

Since walking was no longer any effort for me, I hoped I would be able to run. Now and then. Unfortunately, Kuvalja forbade it. He said people who have problems with damaged cartilage in their vertical pose, whether it is in the spine, hips or knees, should not run, or jump, especially on a hard surface, because the vibrations cause micro-trauma to the cartilage.

"You always have to bear in mind a couple of standard natural variables," Kuvalja told me. "The first is gravity. The second is our weight, our body mass. Third, we want to walk upright. The construction must be upright, and bear the weight. The burden is on the joint cartilage. Each one separately. Each vertebra, the pelvis, hips, knees, ankles, the feet. The shoulder belt, in connection with gravity, has less of a burden, but it is more linked to movement. So, these are the basics. The suspension of a car can take up to five hundred kilos. They get weaker, but you go on driving the same weight. Then they begin to rub on the structure and break parts off. That happens to our joints. The same story. That is why running is not for you, but walking, swimming, cycling are good, because while you are sitting on the bike the weight that would be a burden to your legs if you were running, is transferred to the saddle..."

That is to say, why did I want to run? Walking had long been no effort for me. The first time I made the mistake of stopping walking. In order to get tired, I needed a couple of hours. But who has so many hours? No one. When I stopped walking I started putting on weight, so I started again. You can't go to the mountains every day. Running seemed to be the logical solution. That is, the most attractive of several logical ones.

"Recreational sportsmen are often dependent on pace. But continuity is much more important than intensity. If you get your organism used to some form of effort, and for any reason you are not able to exercise, you lose a tremendous amount of strength. Schwarzenegger is really ripped. Put him in bed. Give him food and drink, but don't let him exercise. His well exercised muscles can lose three per cent of their strength a day. He could pull five hundred Newtons. He would lose fifteen Newtons a day. I can pull one hundred Newtons. And I won't lose even three Newtons. In the end we return to our basic parameters. To carry your own weight you need a minimum, but for his weight, that minimum is much higher. If he doesn't exercise, Schwarzenegger will have problems a lot quicker than you. If you are thirty or forty years old, find yourself a form of exercise that you will be able to do when you are fifty or sixty. Let's say, twice a week, and if possible one that activates all your muscles. Then, if you only play tennis, the same muscles are being activated all the time, and others aren't, so you will have problems. So, different things. Sometimes tennis, sometimes walking, riding a bike, chopping wood... It is not simple, but this is the best way. Look... A farmer doesn't know about squash, skiing, tennis, he has no idea. But a farmer gets up in the morning, drinks his schnapps on an empty stomach. Then his wife makes him coffee. He lights a cigarette, and has a bit of breakfast. And then he goes into the barn to work. He shovels manure, tosses hay, feeds the animals. He has a rest. He goes

Tomislav Birtić

into the field. He loads the tractor, the trailer, he works. Lunch. He has a rest. He does his afternoon shift, and so on, every day. It is balanced. All his muscles are active."

THE DOCTOR SAYS, A BIT OF FAT IS GOOD

Let us recall, on the first day of this story I was unable to walk half a mile. I had to stop. All out of breath. My limit was to walk three, then six miles (five, then ten kilometres). Then I walked eighteen miles (thirty kilometres) in one day. Walking on flat ground was no longer a challenge, so it was a good thing that I began to love mountaineering. Nine miles (fifteen kilometres) on Medvednica, or as we call it in Zagreb, Sljeme, our pet mountain, was no effort for me at all. Four or five hours climbing Risnjak, and the same coming down, was pure joy. Nine hours of very difficult terrain on Biokovo, if we overlook the fact that my knees suffered from the big rocks, wonderful. And now, what can a man over forty do to lose all that flab, so there is nothing to pinch on his hips?

"I wouldn't do that," Kuvalja told me. "If you want a six-pack..."

"... uh, I don't want a six-pack," I interrupted him, "Who could keep that up?"

"Well, if you really want to burn up the fat in precisely defined parts of your body, you can do it, you can work precisely defined muscle groups, to tighten them. You can do that in a gym, but again if you do it under professional supervision."

And then my friend wanted to score a point.

"What is key, what needs to be stressed..." he began.

Tomislav Birtić

"Go on."

"Why are you healthy? You have been climbing hills for years. Because you came to me in time. In time, as soon as the problems began. If you had come later, we would not have managed to restore you, but we would have had to treat you. That is the key difference. People wait. First they are in pain. They put up with it... I had a patient who came after five MRIs of her spine. It hurt, but she never went for treatment. I asked why she had only had images taken. Did she think that the magnet would cure her? Many are almost proud of having had an MRI. And they are happy because they know what is wrong, but they don't have any treatment, they don't do anything. It is very important to see someone as soon as you think something is wrong."

If we think about different generations, and professions, the most at risk are the "office rats," but most people with serious injuries who come to Kuvalja are young, male with a university degree. They used to play a sport, and then their careers took off, seven to eight years of their career... All the same story. The picture of what you used to be able to do remains in your head. You see yourself as a basketball player, you can do anything. You leap over a fence. But that was just what you used to be able to do. The periphery, the executive has lost his strength and coordination, got out of line. And after seven or eight years the young manager has settled his situation at work, whether as the owner or an employee, his family is settled, and he decides he wants to do some sport again. The gang agrees, they are going to shoot some hoops. And they all fall apart. There are hoards of men like that in rehabilitation, says Kuvalja. And these young people, who cost their employers so much, are unfortunately damaged. If they had come for an examination, where the machine shows a deviation of one per cent, they would not have suffered any injury.

Yes... I am one of them. A textbook case. Years and years of a career, then exercise. My muscles at thirty per cent of their desired strength, injury...

EAT TO COMPETE, I ATE LIKE A RUGBY PLAYER. BUT IF I REALLY DID NEED TO EAT IN THE EVENING, THEN FIBRE

I asked the physiotherapist, Alica Fabijanić, who, with Ivo Nuić managed my rehabilitation at the Cybex centre, to create a diet for me – because she looked good. To put it simply, she was slim, and she could lift a stretcher with me on it weighing 253 pounds (115 kilos) with no problem.

"It would have been ideal for you to lose 66 pounds (30 kilos) in a year, and not five months. If you had lost weight as you should, we wouldn't be "hanging out" together today. Actually your body was starved, totally starved. Then your body started to use its reserves. You have a certain percentage of fat which the body will use, and then it will stop. It won't move any more. You can literally stop eating, walk to the end of the world, nearly kill yourself by not eating, but you won't lose any fat. That is, you lose proteins. You started to eat your own muscles. And why ham of all things?! It's pure salt. If only you had eaten some form of veal. But, well, you imagined you needed some form of protein replacement."

"When I was very fat, it was hard for me to get up off a couch. As I lost weight, I was as light as a feather; I got up like a sprinter off the blocks. But later, although I weighed the same, it got harder to get up. So, is that because I was eating my own muscles?"

"Yes. After you got rid of the flab, you started to eat your own proteins. Remember the tests. In some of them your muscles had only thirty per cent strength. So, how could you get up? Not at all. You didn't have strength to control your own body."

"Of all that food science, is there anything that is at least generally accepted, something that would fit in a definition – if you eat that, you won't be wrong?"

"It's like this... Since I work with normal people and with competitive sportsmen and women, I have read loads of books about nutrition. The former national rugby team selector gave me a book called, "Eat to Compete". So, there is a very simple formula in there. A normal breakfast, a bit more fibre for lunch, and proteins for supper. I suggest what we eat, as a national team. They are boys of your size. For some of them your overweight 295 pounds (134 kilos) is their normal weight. For lunch we usually eat fibre food instead of glazed rice, some form of protein, turkey, chicken, veal, perhaps even pork, just enough to ease it down. We were never hungry, no one fainted from exhaustion, which you find in other sportsmen. You, you, in your spirit, never felt hungry. But your organism, when it could no longer use its stores of fat, when there was no longer any way to activate them and get them moving, was hungry and ate your muscles."

"Since I have known you I have been having breakfast, even if I have to force myself. Zu Befehl! I have breakfast. Wasa bars with all and everything, including a third or even half a jar of Kinder Lada. After Cybex I pop into a supermarket, it is about four miles (seven kilometres) to walk to my neighbourhood, I buy fried chicken and Cordon Blue, and cook

Tomislav Birtić

some rice. For supper I have ham, possibly some fruit after eight p.m. And in a week I lose 11 pounds (5 kilos), from 253 to 242 (115 to 110). Next week, if I disturb things just a little, I immediately go back to 253. I have the feeling that due to one single piece of bread that I eat in the evening I go back to 253..."

"Eh, you added bread."

"But if I don't eat something sweet in the morning, but for lunch, the same thing happens, I put the weight back on".

"You have already moved your body closer to rest, that is recovery and depositing."

"So that means sweet things closer to supper, are closer to depositing?"

"That's right."

"Why do the pounds come back so easily?"

"Because that is the way our body, our metabolism, functions. Sugars, simple sugars, and slightly more complex sugars, serve as primary energy sources. Exclusively for muscle contraction. As you get nearer to the end of the day, your muscle activity decreases, and it moves on to consumption in the form of muscle energy, in depositing energy for the next efforts you will make. And where else would it deposit it, but in your "spare tyre"..."

"If I have done everything right, at seven or eight in the evening I have eaten only protein, and then I get so hungry I can't stand it, I have to eat something. Is it OK to eat fruit, or Swiss chard for instance?"

"You can eat Swiss chard, or an apple, anything with lots of fibre."

"Collard greens?"

"Collard greens, Savoy cabbage, bananas..."

"So, if you really have to eat after eight in the evening, to prevent you biting one of your house mates, eat fibre?"

"That's right."

"And you won't put on weight?"

"You won't put on weight. The maths are simple."

"How much would I need to climb or walk to be able to eat however much I want, and not put on weight?"

"Remember that first day on Bjelolasica. That's it."

"In the first phase of weight loss, I stopped drinking beer and hard drinks, but I did not give up wine. I drank wine with water, or separately, wine in one glass and water in another. I even drank a lot of wine and water, but the pounds didn't stick..."

"Beer has bubbles, hard drinks have simple sugars, and that covers everything. So you chose the best thing."

"What is the difference between beer and hard drinks? Is beer a lesser evil than hard drinks?"

"Hard drinks are exclusively short sugars. Hard drinks dehydrate you. At least beer leaves your body quite quickly."

"That means, if someone really loves hard drinks, they should force themselves to drink two litres of water after downing a few?"

"Before they drink, not after. So it comes out more quickly."

"The gang invites you out, and you say, "Give me a minute so I can drink two litres of mineral water"..." I laughed.

"Still water. CO2 binds sugars."

"Well if you have to drink for some reason, the best thing to drink is wine – red wine?"

Tomislav Birtić

"It doesn't matter if it is white or red, but don't take dessert wine, because it is sweet. But we need to change your style of training. Put you on a bicycle to burn up the fat you have left. Activity should be light, at a moderate pace, but long lasting. It has to last more than an hour and fifteen minutes, even an hour and a half to use fat."

So, another chapter.

ALL FLUSHED AFTER WALKING ONE MILE – COMPETITIVE SPORTSMAN. CLIMBED A MOUNTAIN WITH NO EFFORT – RECREATIONAL SPORTSMAN

"Some say thirty minutes, some forty five, so you say an hour and fifteen or even thirty minutes to burn fat. Is that connected to the pulse, so your pulse has to be above 120-130 to lose weight, or does it have to last for an hour and a half, regardless of your pulse?" I asked the physiotherapist.

"If you want to become a scientist and get involved in training, you have left the zone of recreational sport, now you are in the zone of training, and you will be like Lance Armstrong. You will weigh your food, and everything will be determined by your pulse. But it is not absolutely necessary. It is enough to have moderate physical activity for a longer period of time. Why must it be more than an hour? Because if you train for only half an hour, the moment when you are on your bicycle and you stop at the traffic lights, you put down your foot and wait for the green light, is enough for your body to stop using fat and start doing something else."

"Like a child I used to question the minute rest. What was that for?! Who can rest for half a minute or a minute?! But, when we are walking we are tired, but we don't stop. You have to stop at the traffic lights because they are red, and while waiting for the red to change to green, I rest enough to walk for the next half an hour without strain."

"Yes! That's what I am saying!"

"But, now, is it OK to take a minute's rest? Or should you deny your body that if you want to lose weight?"

"While you are losing weight, you should not be so tired that you need a minute's break. If you need a minute's break, you are no longer losing weight, but you are beginning to train."

"Does it confuse your organism if it was just recreational sport but you got really fit and actually became like a competitive sportsman, and then you got unfit again and went back to being like a recreational sportsman again?"

"You need to define "recreation"."

"Fast walking, five miles (eight and a half kilometres) an hour?"

"That is training. That is not recreation."

"At the beginning of the story I was not capable of walking a few hundred metres. I would get so tired I had to sit down..."

"... That is pure training," she interrupted me.

"Training?"

"Yes. That is not a weight losing process."

"But I could hardly move. It wasn't fast walking. How could that waddling be sport?"

"Don't mix chalk and cheese. You had 295 pounds (134 kilos) of unfunctional body mass, which exerted additional pressure on your heart and blood vessels."

"So for me any movement was like training?"

"Yes! For you any movement was like training. And what's more, you were smoking three packets a day."

"The mountain route on which I had to stop at least twice before coming to Cybex, I went up without stopping. Although part of it was under deep snow, so it took more effort to pull my legs out of the snow than to climb. I only stopped for a few seconds, because I was thirsty. I had to have a drink. Was that training or recreation?"

"Well, now you have gone back to recreation, because you have sufficiently trained your body, so climbing the mountain along that route had started to be recreation. It is now too easy for you."

"But I got really out of breath," I really wanted my activity to be counted as a serious sport after all.

"The right words. You got really out of breath, but you didn't need to stop, catch your breath, pull yourself together, like you did when you first went walking and then climbing. That means you are now a recreational sportsman."

"Do I need, in order to burn up my fat completely, to do anaerobic exercises, and combine them two or three times a week with aerobic exercises?"

"Noooo. You don't need to do anaerobic exercises. We only need to maintain your condition. If you only did aerobic exercises, you would burn up your fat. No problem."

"Let's translate that into real life. I live near a swimming pool..."

"Don't start swimming. First you have to realize that water makes your body lighter. That means, you have to swim for two hours to use up the fat."

"Forget it. Two hours! So we can forget swimming immediately!"

"The other thing is, your technique is doubtful, the question is whether you would move your arms and legs to activate your muscles. I swim in the summer. My normal phase is two and a half mile (four

Tomislav Birtić

kilometres) a day. That is long distance. However I do sprints of fifty metres in the last half of mile. After that I feel like an aeroplane."

"So it seems: OK, swim, but don't count it as losing weight."

"Thank you for saying that. You won't lose much weight by swimming."

"Is tennis good?"

"Come on, please, just go and injure yourself... Realistically, you should do something that fulfils you, for which it is no effort to leave your flat and go there. If tennis is what you like doing, do it! There is no need to look for a new sport. But, now you are in serious danger of injury, so you shouldn't play tennis."

"Nordic walking?"

"Absolutely!"

"How far does one need to walk a day or a week to lose weight?"

"How far can you walk?"

"As far as you like!"

"Then walk for an hour and a half a day, at four miles (seven kilometres) an hour, and that is it. First we will make your heart work as it should. Then, it is time to get rid of those other deposits, from the insides of your blood vessels, and that would be it. I stress, when losing weight, the aim is to do something you like, something that suits you. Otherwise you will give up and the weight will come back, the yo-yo effect."

TERRIBLE MISTAKE – I STOPPED WALKING

And so, and it was really stupid, I declared walking to be uneconomical, compared with mountain climbing. Who would walk six miles (ten kilometres) every day, or at least ten thousand steps, when it involves absolutely no effort? And again, to walk fifteen miles (twenty-five kilometres) every day – no one has that much time. I couldn't run because neither my ankles nor my knees could stand it after twenty years' break. In the end I said that mountain climbing once a week or twice a month was enough to achieve my goals.

In a flash I went from 242 to 260 pounds (110 to 118 kilos). Fortunately, when I made the terrible mistake of stopping exercising every day, at least I still didn't use public transport, so I weighed 264 pounds (120 kilos) for a short time, but nothing more than that. But 253 pounds (115 kilos) was also the limit that I couldn't break through.

The torture began. I still didn't know then that it is hard to change a trend. I made the bitter discovery that you cannot lose 5 pounds when you want, in two hours of exercise.

Tomislav Birtić

DUKAN. IT'S NOT FOR ME

Every so often there is an article in the paper about the Dukan diet. Chance would have it that I read about it in Jutarnji list. By the book. A French doctor came up with a diet rich in proteins, which will get you to your ideal weight. The Dukan diet – the "secret" of French skinniness. Today more than a million and a half French people swear by it, and recently stars such as Gisele Bundchen and Jennifer Lopez have signed up to it. They emphasize its long-lasting results as its best characteristic. The last phase of the diet lasts until the end of your life, and the only requirement is that you eat only proteins one day a week. No question, a great introduction to the subject.

The article wrote that Dr. Pierre Dukan came up with the diet completely by accident, while he was working as a neurosurgeon. His friend asked him to recommend a diet, but without leaving out meat. Dukan told him to eat nothing but protein for five days, and to drink only water. The doctor and the friend were shocked – the friend lost 9 pounds (4.5 kilos). Another five days eating only proteins and drinking only water, and he lost another 6 pounds (3 kilos). The excited Dukan left neurosurgery and for the next thirty-five years he researched and developed his diet.

The diet is in four phases. It starts with a sudden loss of weight in a few days, when you are not allowed to eat anything but protein. Depending on how much weight you want to lose, this "attack phase" can last from one day to ten days. You then add vegetables in unlimited quantities. In that period you should lost a 2 pounds (kilo) a week. After reaching your ideal weight, or the weight Dr. Dukan recommends (I read in Jutarnji list that there is a test on his internet site which will calculate your ideal weight), you begin the phase of "consolidation" in which you slowly introduce again all those foods which you avoided during the first two phases, like fruit, bread, cheese, pasta... In that period there is no weight loss, nor gain. And then – the rest of your life, in which you can eat anything, but one day a week has to be just protein. He suggests Thursdays, and most of his followers do what he says.

The next day I bought Jutarnji list again to read more detailed instructions. It said that if I want to lose more than 39 pounds (18 kilos), the first phase should last at least seven days. I weighed myself, 262 pounds (119 kilos). I wanted to weigh less than 220 pounds (100 kilos).

And, just as the doctor said, I ate only protein, and drank water. It is impossible to describe how hard that was for me. I lasted for four days of chicken, veal, beef, eggs, cheese, fish, and then seeking a new taste to ease my pain, on the sixth day I went to the shop for some salmon. It is true, I lost 8 pounds (4 kilos), but I gave up. I did not make it to the second phase.

I stress that this is not a criticism of Dukan's method, and in the end, who am I to argue with him? But it was not for me. Later I bought his book, but, with all

Tomislav Birtić

due respect, either the diet is not for me, or I am not for the Dukan diet.

SIX AND A HALF HOURS' WALKING – 6 POUNDS (3 KILOS) MORE?

It rained for two weeks, two weekends. In the end, there was a little sun on the second Sunday. I longed for the hills so much, that I decided to spend the entire day in the woods. To make up for what I had missed.

From the tram to the foot of the climb it is twenty minutes' easy walking. This time I had a camera around my neck, so I walked at a pace to stop it banging. I kept stopping to take pictures of other mountain walkers or the countryside. Three hours, that means the hardest seven hundred metres' climb to the top. But this time, I didn't eat anything at the top and come back to town by bus, but I went down to mountain hut, got changed and had lunch, then walked the entire route I usually rode. A total of six and a half hours' walking. A pleasant effort, pure, indescribable pleasure.

In the morning before I set out, and at about one, about an hour before lunch, I ate a piece of chocolate. I had fried chicken for lunch, with potatoes and cabbage salad, and at home in the evening I ate a sandwich. The next day I weighed 6 pounds (3 kilos) more! What a shock! I walk for two or three hours, and the next day I regularly weigh at least 2 pounds (kilo) less, but after six and a half hours walking I weighed 6 pounds (3 kilos) more.

I told my Doctor, Željko Šućur all this in a message.

Tomislav Birtić

"Expected! Water! Eat in moderation, drink large quantities of water, your weight falls in a couple of days. For sure," Šućur reassured me.

It was just as Šućur said.

HERBALIFE IS IT,
I TAKE HERBALIFE EVERY DAY

A friend of a friend, my acquaintance, lives in London. Like many others, he longs to own property in West London. A small flat, a really small flat, costs several million pounds in that area. Wanting to explain why I take Herbalife, I told him... Imagine your dream came true. You have a huge flat in West London, and several billion pounds in the bank, or dollars or whatever. So, you can eat whatever you like. Where will you get your carrots? I could see in his eyes that he was beginning to understand. Well, I will get carrots delivered by helicopter to the roof or garden of my house. Every day until the end of my life, so I can eat the best, I will pay two hundred pounds a kilo for the best carrots. But, where will they be delivered from? In contrast to my mother, whose garden is just a few steps away from the kitchen table, and who has been eating healthy food since she can remember, someone who lives in West London, you could say, is in a less favourable position. Now, after we have agreed that a millionaire or billionaire from West London will eat healthy food (perhaps not like my mother, but still healthy), the question is what will poor people eat, or the middle class? An apple that has eight times less nutritional value than twenty or thirty years ago? Vegetables and fruit that ripen on shelves? What kind of meat? So, there we are, that is why I use food supplements. I chose Herbalife. As a teenager I came across Fleetwood Mac, and I have

Tomislav Birtić

been listening to them ever since. The first food supplement I heard of was Herbalife. I liked it, it helped me, and that was that. Perhaps I am the only person it helps in the entire world. Perhaps I only imagine it; perhaps it doesn't have any effect even on me. But there you are, I take it every day.

I have to say that I am in double conflict of interests. I am a shareholder in Herbalife, and a distributor. It doesn't matter how much, but I am obliged to say that I make money selling Herbalife products. And I have to say, that the company Herbalife had no part in my venture, nor in the making of my book, and I have to say that this is just my experience.

Now we have got that out of the way, I will say that before Herbalife stopped being an experiment for me, I experimented with Herbalife for three years. In the first year, I lost weight, and then due to a poor diet, which was not the fault of Herbalife, I put that weight back on again. For the entire second year of the experiment, without Herbalife in my diet, I put on weight, or I barely, with extreme effort, managed to maintain my weight. In the third year, with the help of Blanka Perše, whom I will introduce to you in a minute, so with Blanka, a metabolic balance, and Herbalife, finally, after seven years' wandering, I found my way. I lost weight, I feel great, and I am not putting the weight back on.

The story goes like this. I came out of the building where I live and met someone I know at the bus stop. He asked me where I was going, I told him I was going to walk around the lake, to try to lose weight. He then suggested I try to lose weight using Herbalife. However funny it sounds, the key was when he said, "You have to take in a total of one hundred and fourteen nutrients every day." If he had said fifty or hundred I would not have batted an eyelid. But, one hundred and fourteen – that sounded a bit like science. My experience tells me, where the superiority of the spirit over matter ends, the human need for science begins.

In a few minutes, in the time I spent keeping him company until his bus came along, he told me too much to remember it all. But the key was this: although he was a former sportsman, and former sportsmen routinely get fat, he looked like he did while he was still playing. Perfect.

A day later I was staring at Omron's diagnostic scales, a piece of apparatus like bathroom scales, just like I have had all my life, but the difference is that to the left and right of the screen it has three metal plates, and as you weigh yourself you hold some sort of handles out in front of yourself. The machine measures your body mass, then your body mass index, your subcutaneous fat, your visceral fat, or the fat inside your abdomen, around your organs, and it measures your muscles and base metabolism, that is the number of calories your body uses in a state of rest.

I stood on the scales, barefoot. Dressed, I weight 266 pounds (120.9 kilos). Fat 37.4. At the age of 40, the normal zone is 11 to 22. From 22 to 28 is excess, and above 28 it is horrible. The aim is 22. Visceral fat – around the organs: 13. He told me that anything above 10 is a problem (wow! What would that machine have measured when I weighed 266 pounds and hardly moved?). The aim was no more than 9. Muscles 27.5, and 37 was desirable. Body mass index

– 30.4. The healthy zone is from 18.5 to 25, above 30 is obese. So, the aim is 25.

Since I wanted to lose at least 44 pounds (20 kilos), he suggested I had a Herbalife shake for breakfast and dinner, and for lunch I could eat whatever I liked, with no limitations. Specifically, for lunch I should definitely eat some form of protein. Something with feathers. Turkey, chicken, or perhaps veal. Or fish. Avoid red meat, because, he said, the remains of red meat sit in your digestive system for up to six months, in your intestines. So, if you do eat red meat, you need to eat a lot of fibre.

"Let's say, two sarma (a sour cabbage roll with meat and rice) for lunch, with a little bit of bread. Is that it?" I asked him.

"Yes. With this programme you can eat three to four sarma with no problem. As you like."

"So, one day two sarma, the next day peas with noodles and chicken, the third day spinach with a can of..."

"Try to eat salad for lunch."

And so that is what my days looked like on Herbalife.

Immediately in the morning, when I woke up, I would make myself a Thermojetics tea. A teaspoonful in half a litre of warm water. I would drink it with two compressed fibres, Fiber and Herbs.

Breakfast, twenty minutes after the Thermojetics, a shake. Three to four spoonfuls in two to two and a half decilitres of milk. Or juice, my mentor told me, but to start with I only made the shake with milk, later with soya milk. I drank the shake slowly, I really enjoyed it.

Two hours later I had a snack. Fruit or a Herbalife protein bar. With a glass of water.

About two hours after that came lunch. I did not deny myself anything. Chicken, turkey, fish, very, very rarely tofu, low-fat cheese. And always a big salad. With my lunch a Thermojetics and Fiber and Herbs. (If I could not avoid a business dinner in the evening I would have a shake for lunch, and I would eat for supper whatever I would have had for lunch.)

About three hours after lunch, an apple or a protein bar.

In the evening a shake, and fibre.

My mentor added that I could drink a shake if necessary after training, and I should drink four and a half litres of water a day (a litre for every 55 pounds (25 kilos) of weight), and if I had symptoms of detoxification, like headaches, constipation, strong thirst, I should hold on and drink more water so the toxins would leave my body as soon as possible.

Well....

The shake would keep me feeling full for several hours. As they say, I couldn't believe that someone could be full from eating three spoonfuls of powder and a little soya milk.

As for Thermojetics... I went on a business trip. Fortunately by car. If not at every, then at every other service station, we had to stop so I could go to the toilet. For two weeks my skin itched, mostly my chest, arms and back. But as I said, after two weeks it stopped.

The best part of the story is that while I was resting due to an injury, I lost so much weight it was crazy, 8 pounds (4 kilos) a month, 4 pounds (2 kilos)...

Tomislav Birtić

Encouraged by the results, I reinforced the Herbalife programme with multivitamin tables, minerals and omega. The luckier ones amongst us would say that they had never had so many compliments about their skin in their lives. But I had never had any compliments on my skin. Now women started complimenting me routinely. They were amazed and asked me what I used. Women who had never noticed me before, or who would say hello out of politeness, would now say "Kisses! See you!" at the end of coffee break. (My best friend from high school said that research had shown that women always choose men with a stronger immune system than their own. Specifically, in that research they were only able to investigate a square centimetre of the man's face. The rest was covered in cloth. By seeing, touching, smelling that small piece of skin, they had to say who in their opinion would be the best partner for life, to advance the species. And, as she said, they all chose the men with a stronger immune system than they had themselves. That would be my layman's explanation for my sudden popularity amongst women who had never even noticed me before...)

The down side of the story is that when I recovered from my injury, I was still on two shakes and lunch, even when I was doing hard training. For instance, an hour and a half of Cybex, and another hour and more walking, mountaineering at the weekends. For a while I would keep going on the rhythm of a shake for breakfast, a protein bar as a snack, a big lunch, a protein bar for another snack and a shake for supper. But, using calories as I was, sooner or later I would be so hungry that I would eat something else, outside the regime, and my body, furiously hungry, overcome with panic, would take that and store it so efficiently as fat, that it was incredible. I had the feeling that my body created a 2 pounds of fat out of a slice of bread.

I concluded that static types, as we call them, office rats, achieve their aims using the method suggested by the man who recommended Herbalife to me, but different rules apply to sportsmen.

Whatever the case, in the second year of the experiment I did not take Herbalife, and from 242 pounds (110 kilos) my weight rose to 264 pounds (120 kilos) in a jiffy. The jiffy took about three months, and then I struggled, by walking and keeping a strict control on my calorie intake. The experiment showed that there is no healthy life without a dietary supplement. I admit that someone may win a Nobel Prize proving otherwise, I admit that this is already common knowledge, but I can't imagine my own diet without any supplements.

In the third year of my experiment with Herbalife, the shake was no longer breakfast for me, to replace a meal, but an addition to breakfast, and most often for dinner too. I say, "most often", because I would often have one after lunch as a dessert. I would go into the mountains with my friends, and after beans and sausages, or stew, or ham and sour cabbage, I take or, if you like, drink a shake instead of a cake. At home I sometimes make it with a little milk, so it is thick like blancmange. It is tasty, sweet and healthy, mounds of protein, vitamins and minerals. So, concluding that a key requirement for losing weight is feeling full, adjusting my intake of nutrients and calories to my physical activity – I was saved. That was when my final rebirth began, which became my life style.

Tomislav Birtić

Again, I stress. I am a Herbalife shareholder and a distributor. I stress that I am a layman, that nothing in this book has the force of scientific research, I emphasize that I cannot even guarantee that the sun will rise tomorrow, let alone that anyone will lose weight after reading about the path I took. But, over the years I have tried various Herbalife products on myself. After long aerobic activity I take a Rebuild Endurance drink, and after exercising on the Cybex machine, whose goal is to increase muscle mass, I take Rebuild Strength. If the measurements show that my muscles are weaker, I sometimes add a spoonful of protein to the shake. For my body to have sufficient carbohydrates and minerals for hard work, such as difficult climbs for instance, and so that it won't start consuming muscles, and to enable it simply to melt fats, I take H3O. A wonderful isotonic. I take Fiber and Herbs twice a year for a month. Always in January, after breaking all the rules of dieting over the holidays, and on my summer holidays, because my discipline breaks down a little then. I take vitamins and minerals in the winter, because there are no fresh vegetables or fruit (in that order) from my mum's garden at that time. I drink Thermojectics very often, and if I don't drink Thermojetics, then I drink green tea. And so on.

THE VERVITA OR HUROM JUICER, THAT IS, FOOD IS THE BEST COSMETIC, PART TWO

On the subject of my skin... In the little more than the seven years I spent experimenting on myself before publishing this book, I only received compliments about my skin in two periods. The first was after I started following an intense Herbalife programme, and the second after three months of drinking cold, freshly prepared juices made from vegetables and fruit grown by my parents.

I drank juice from a juicer for the first time as a child. I was ten or maybe a little older. My parents have an orchard and a vegetable garden, so they bought a juicer. What can I say...? I hope that if I have children, the advertisements will be dramatically different than when I was a child. That is, although my parents were careful, and the first juice they made me was from carrots, that is, it was sweet, I believe that that juice stood no chance against the food advertised on television. What's more, it took ages to clean the juicer. It was quickly removed from the kitchen and put in some cupboard, where it was least in the way.

Years later, when I was trying to live a healthy life, I bought one of those food processors. They chop, squeeze juice, grate, all kinds of things. I wouldn't even have thought of buying it if my sister, to whom I had recommended the VerVita juicer, which is known as Hurom elsewhere in the world, had not told me

Tomislav Birtić

that she already had not only a juicer but also a food processor, which I had given her.

Anyhow, what I want to say is... My friend suggested that I should drink cold juices. Then, just to change the subject without offending him, I told him that it was a great idea, that it must be wonderful, but I really could not be bothered to wash the juicer every time. But he didn't give up. He said that the juicer had a great design, that it had only a few parts, and he could take it apart and wash it in only two minutes. Again, really more so I wouldn't hurt his feelings than the fact that I gave any kind of credence to the juicer, I let him tell me everything he wanted about cold, freshly squeezed juices.

And he said... Who could eat ten apples? He didn't know anyone who could. But anyone can drink the juice of ten apples. He went on to say that everything of any value in fruit and vegetables is in the juice. The pulp, the fibre is disposed of through the other hole in the juicer, so he dehydrates it and makes crackers out of it, healthy biscuits. The key, he said, is that the part of the juicer that presses the vegetables and fruit goes round very slowly, so that it does not create a high temperature, which can destroy the nutrients.

He invited me to his place, and he and his girlfriend made me juice from various vegetables and fruit. I laughed like mad at how simple it all was. The most time, but not too much, was taken up washing and cutting the ingredients. And you can't throw them in the juicer as quickly as it makes the juice. In the end he took it apart and washed it in front of me. It really did take less than two minutes. The next day he took me to a shop to buy one.

The first juice I made was from apples. Just apples. And I really liked it. It was very, very tasty. The next one I made was from two savoy cabbage leaves, and some apples. It was, of course, green, greener than Ireland, but sweet. Fantastic. For a few days I experimented, I learned how many leaves I could put in the juice, for it still to be sweet. In a few days I had learned the process itself, and then the festival began. My parents brought me two huge bags full of vegetables and fruit.

Four cabbages, let's say eight savoy cabbage leaves, two medium-sized beetroots, three apples and three pears – fantastic. A bit of celery, two parsley roots, three carrots, a small cup of chokeberries, beetroot, apples and pears – fantastic. Carrots, parsley root, parsnip, celeriac, peppers, savoy cabbage, apples and pears – heaven on earth. A quarter of a head of cabbage, grapes, apples – super. I combined and combined, first of all amazed at how a litre of juice can keep you as full as supper or lunch. And, as I said, again women kept asking me if, like a caveman, I had become a metrosexual, since my skin had become so fine, and even photo-shopped women from magazines didn't have such a good complexion.

But before I turn to my holy grail, which I had been looking for for almost seven years, before I introduce you to Blanka and metabolic balance, a little about Herbalife's competitors. Of course they didn't change my opinion about Herbalife, but I learned a lot about nutrition.

Tomislav Birtić

"IT IS NOT ABOUT LOSING WEIGHT, BUT PEOPLE NEED TO CHANGE THEIR LIVES"

In Medikor's display window I saw a pot almost identical to the one used for Herbalife shakes. It said Spiru-Tein on it. I went into the shop and started to talk to a woman in a white overall. As students we used to joke that if you see a man in a white coat, he obviously thinks he is a scientist.

"Doctors say that they can advise their patients only in the same way they would advise their mother or sister..."

"That's right," she said.

"And would you advise me to take your Spiru-Tein or Herbalife?"

"Of course I would recommend Spiru-Tein."

I introduced myself, said I was writing a book, and that I would like to interview her. She replied that the nutritionist Branimir Dolibašić was authorized for that. I left her my mobile number and asked her to pass the message on to him. He called me in less than half an hour. The next day we were already sitting in his office, and joking how the fierce competitors, Herbalife and Spiru-Tein, had stores right next to each other, and their head offices were at the same address, on the same stairwell. I told him that I didn't have time nor pages to interview all Herbalife's market competitors, so, you see, I had chosen him to represent, not just his own company, but all the other competitors, that is, it would be ideal if he could rise far above economics, and focus on people, on each person, as if they were his son, brother or father. My impression is the Dolibašić was more than successful at this.

Let's go.

"What we are trying to do should not be called losing weight," Dolibašić began, as a nutritionist, the head of a diet advisory centre. "We shouldn't say how to lose weight as easily as possible, or how to beat the kilos. Spiru-Tein is not something that will make people lose weight, but they will lose weight when they change their lives. We can thank Spiru-Tein in the most fantastic words. But kilos are not a one-way street, or a machine you put a coin into, and a bucket comes out and you are saved. That is not how it works."

"How can a lay person find his way in the plethora of different proteins, food and dietary supplements? Let's say, there are five Nobel Prize winners, sitting around a table. They all received their Nobel Prizes for nutrition and they all say, about the other four, that they are amazed that they even passed their degrees, that they talk a load of rubbish... How can a layman find his way? What should he choose?"

"Ah, that is a hard question."

"I don't think it is so hard."

"...!" a mixture of amazement and expectation on Dolibašić's face.

"They will choose whatever Messi is advertising," I said. It was a joke, because Messi advertised Herbalife, but perhaps it is a universal truth. As a child I used to eat Nestle chocolate because I had heard that Borg advertised it. If he had advertised eating dirt, as a boy, I would have eaten it, convinced that it would help me win Wimbledon.

"We live in that kind of society and time," Dolibašić shrugged his shoulders.

"But, what can you tell me, why should I buy your protein, and not some other brand, which a body builder tells me is the only one that does not clog up my kidneys? We are not talking about Herbalife nor Spiru-Tein here, nor about any specific product, but about principles."

"Let us go back to the beginning of the problem. If you want to lose weight, you don't need Spiru-Tein. You need will and discipline. Spiru-Tein is something that makes that path easier. When we reach a stable weight one day, we can keep taking Spiru-Tein like an old friend. I want people to know about Spiru-Tein in that story, so they know there is a choice. I think it is a fantastic product. It also tastes really good. But it is also functional, it brings real benefits."

"Doctors told me that I was using up my muscles instead of fat because of my poor diet. Would Spiru-Tein have helped me, or, to be honest about all these products, would any isolated protein have helped stop my muscles being damaged?"

"Yes. Any protein which has some biological value would have performed its function in that situation. When someone sets out to lose weight, he is like a ship going out into a storm. Actually, a person consciously creates the storm, he chooses the path towards the storm. What should he do when the boat begins to rock? There are efficient or crude solutions, and there are also sophisticated or better solutions. In that sense, Spiru-Tein is a sophisticated weapon. Not just as a source of protein, but much more than that. When a piece of chicken is compared to a Spiru-Tein meal, then the Spiru-Tein meal is attributed with various splendours and useful nutritional functions, which a piece of chicken does not have, and a Spiru-Tein meal may have an equal amount of protein. But I say, losing weight is a complex process, it is not just a matter of proteins."

And now the fun really begins, Dolibašić's philosophy of food, his holistic approach.

"WE HAVE ALL THE PREDISPOSITIONS WE NEED TO LIVE AS KINGS USED TO LIVE, BUT WE DON'T HAVE THE BRAINS"

"Is it true that on many farms they give animals steroids in order to..."

"... they give them steroids and antibiotics," Dolibašić interrupted me.

"OK, antibiotics, so the animals wouldn't get sick before they are slaughtered, and steroids, I suppose, as I have read, so the farmers can get not one or two feeding cycles but four in the same period of time. It seems that in food today there are substances which weaken people's immunity and make them fat, whilst some people have told me that in the apples that city people usually buy today there are eight times fewer nutritional ingredients than twenty or whatever years ago. What I mean is, if we don't have the same nutrients as our forebears, they at least didn't have to defend themselves from the food they were eating..."

"That is the paradox of modern times, and it is, at least partially, true. But it is wrong to think about food solely by just transferring the food our ancestors ate into the modern age. Life before was not like it is now. People used to sleep eight or nine hours. In the evening they would go to sleep, they did not waste their nerves by watching television, but the evening was a time for relaxing. Every evening was a wellness evening. Today we ride everywhere. We go by car, we ride in lifts, we ride in trams. We do not do physically demanding work. We have learned to be passive in every possible way, and this passivity uses up our knees, our elbows, our feet, our fingers... and in the end our bodies call us to account. In our forties! Whoops! Our spine is no longer what it was. Why? Our modern way of life is to blame. Before people didn't need yoga, stretching, Pilates, private trainers, but they had hoes, and they stretched by getting things down from a shelf in the larder. Today we actually have all we need to live as only kings were able to live before, but we don't have the brains for it. We are not intelligent enough regarding food, that is, we let advertising tell us what to eat. A lot of advertisements are nothing more than instructions on how we should live, and those instructions are very, very primitive. They tell us: Buy this and you will be happy in life! Thirty years ago it was OK to advertise cigarettes, today that is forbidden. Some prominent nutritionists think that many of today's advertisements could be banned in their present form in the near future because they are advertising things that are just as harmful as smoking. They are advertising bad food. Responsibility! We make trashy food, but we don't care. Unfortunately, people are not sensible enough to choose healthy food."

"I wouldn't say that sense is the only problem. In Manhattan every day several million people come down from their skyscrapers for lunch. Food costs from one dollar, for the worst kind of hot dog, to forty dollars, which is what I paid for a good meal. A dollar, or forty? People say, "Who doesn't pay the whore, pays the doctor". In this case, who doesn't pay for healthy food (and many don't pay, not because they don't have the brains, but because they don't have the money), pays the doctor. Or they can't even pay

Tomislav Birtić

the doctor because they don't have any money. What can people do? Where should they eat? What should they eat?"

"For you to find or prepare a really healthy meal by yourself, you don't need more than thirty kunas (abut five dollars) per meal. Per meal! And if you are lucky, per day. However, yes! You need to think about it, to make an effort. And you also need a bit of time. To look, and for instance when you are travelling, to plan ahead where you can buy a healthy apple, or walnuts in a town... If there are no shops with good food in the town, before you travel you have to buy healthy food where you live, and take the food with you."

"Are food supplements actually our salvation? If I can't get an apple like I ate when I was a child, which had as many nutritious ingredients as eight apples from my store today, I can take vitamins that have been taken from an apple which a farmer claims was grown like the apples from my childhood."

"That won't save you. Yes, vitamins are good. Yes, vitamins have a function. But they are not a magic solution, and they do not exclude food. The best vitamin products imitate food. But let us go back to the beginning. Hunters and gatherers search for food every day. The leaders of tribes, kings, are brought food at the table, but all the rest of us have to search for our food ourselves. Today's fruit is classified, but those classes unfortunately do not include nutritional value, but weight, free of spots... Americans, for example, prescribed long age by law that all the important information had to be included in food declarations, such as sodium, fat and cholesterol content, so people really have no excuse if they don't know if they are buying food that will kill them. Americans have also made a huge effort to educate their people. We can really congratulate them on that. There are a million ways for someone to get information on health there, without someone trying to sell you something, but in a true desire for people to be healthy. The fact that the nation is overweight has forced them into this. In Europe the authorities are nowhere near so agile concerning obesity, we believe that our tradition will save us."

"OK... Let's say that the god of healthy food comes down to Earth and tells me what the recommended amounts are of which substances, just like that, just for me. And now, I take in all the substances I need, precisely as much as I need. Now I need calories. If I have taken in all the milligrams I need, I still can't live if I don't have dekagrams and kilograms – calories. How can I save myself, so the calories won't do me any harm? So it is not a chicken, drugged up with steroids and antibiotics, a plastic apple..."

"Here again, it is best to go back to the beginning. We have to learn to feed ourselves and we have to learn to find our food. When things get out of control, protein meals like Spiru-Tein are a lifebelt. There is no substitute for food which people have to eat. There is no guru, no coach, who will remove the need for food, or sit every day like an angel on your shoulder and tell you what to do. You have to gain that knowledge for yourself. Before the choice was simple: healthy food or death. Because there was not enough food. What was the average diet like in Croatia only one hundred years ago? Maize, rye, potatoes, vegetables, milk products. Meat was extremely expensive. For the common farmer, it was incredibly expensive to

Tomislav Birtić

kill a chicken or a cow. There were eggs sometimes, there was milk, which was also quite expensive, so people looked for ways to conserve it, to make it last as long as possible. That means, people ordered their food according to sources of protein, and the daily aim was to provide a source of starch as the main source of energy. There were always enough vegetables and fruit, and people always took care that they would be the basis of their everyday diet. People always cooked peas, beans, porridge in advance, or baked bread. This was the energy which drove people. Fats were scarce, there were not as many as their physical requirements demanded. And people were slim, although they ate pure pork fat, because they burned up that fat, with no remainder. Because they worked hard every day. That element of physical activity must be re-introduced into modern life. OK, but we live in a city. What can we do? Fitness, running, riding a bike. We still do not live in a destroyed environment, without an inch of greenery, we have places to go. We have to make use of them, and every day make time for good physical activities. That is the portion of vitamins people are lacking today," he made his point.

"DIET, WALKING, STRENGTHING, BALANCE STRETCHING, PSYCHE – THE PROBLEM SOLVED"

"In my research... I walked home from work every day. While I was walking every day, everything was fine. But after I had walked eighteen miles (thirty kilometres) in one day, after walking no longer made me tired, I stopped walking every day. So, walking didn't make me tired, and I did not dare to run because due to my age and years of a sedentary lifestyle, my body was out of line, my ankles and knees would not have been able to take running. So I started to climb. But, who goes up Sljeme (the mountain to the north of Zagreb) every day?! It takes an hour just to get there and back. And climbing stairs every day.... that was too monotonous, too dull. That was when my weight loss stopped, and as soon as I stopped watching what I ate, even a little, I quickly put the weight back on. Fortunately I could easily get it off again. And then I started to jog. And it was instant sweat! When I was climbing I would start to sweat after about fifteen minutes, but when I started jogging it was immediate. I was thrilled. Is the solution for me to jog every day now?"

"No. We have to go back to the beginning again. Diet and the human body have to be seen holistically. This means, diet and activity are inseparable. There is not one, best form of exercise. My blood boils when I read newspapers and popular books which oversimplify things. Of course, sometimes we have to make things simple so people can understand. But when someone does it who doesn't understand it themself, then the result can be incomprehensible tripe. Unfortunately, this is how it is with most popular diets. It sounds great when they say you lose weight only by eating certain food or doing special exercises, but it is actually ridiculous, because people work really hard for a while, but then the weight just comes back again. In relation to exercise: walking – yes. But walking is only one form of exercise. Walking is an aerobic form of using energy. Regarding walking, you have got it, you deserve all honours, diplomas, expressions of praise, medals, whatever. However, strength is a different matter. The third thing is balance. And the fourth is stretching. Those four things need to be practised equally every day."

"I tried standing on one leg for a minute, with my arms stretched out in front of me, a little to the side. I would watch Bloomberg or CNBC, those financial channels have a clock at the bottom of the screen, so I could time one minute. I was surprised at how much a man can sweat..."

"Yes... You can practise strength in the gym, but I, for example, have been exercising for three years now, carrying my son, who now weighs forty four pounds (twenty kilos). And stretching? A mat on the floor, and exercise. Any good fitness coach knows how to do it."

"You mean, if I add exercises to my walking, for balance, strength and stretching, I will have solved all my problems?"

"If you do it every day, you will have resolved the problem of physical exercise. All that remains is diet. Proteins are the only thing that must be brought under control. Yes, that is a large part of the balance, but far from the whole. Also, you have to adjust your fat intake. Fats must never be left out of your diet. They can be reduced, but never left out. Your body must have fat. We are physiologically built to be practically dependent on it. It is so important to our body that it will produce fat itself if we don't take it in. So our body doesn't need to find a way to produce fat itself, we make its work easier by taking in fat with our food. There is an important exception here. There is a kind of fat which it can't produce itself. This is the famous omega fats. Omega 3 and omega 6. To function well, our body needs a little bit of these omegas every day. Well, the question is now, how to get them in our food, and which food? There are people who reduce or throw out fat when they are on a diet, and then their body looks for fat. This is the cry of a metabolism denied. If people are on a diet, if they are refraining from fat, it is really difficult. The food industry was ready and waiting to make it more difficult, so today we have milk that has almost no fat in it. We have an abundance of light milk, which, apart from a reduced percentage of fat, also has no omega. That is why people need to be educated about their own diet, and every day they need to look for food which has a source of omega for their needs."

"Should they buy tablets?"

"OK, they can buy capsules. If they can't get, let's say, walnuts or fish every day, they should buy omega in capsules or good quality, cold-pressed oil, to be sure they get the omega they need every day."

"My parents sometimes send me walnuts from Slavonia, and I can't stop eating them. Does that mean my body is screaming out for omega?"

Tomislav Birtić

"It needs omega, that is it. That is the cry of your body."

Now we come to the part of the book prepared by Dolibašić himself. That is to say, when I sent him the chapter he contributed to for authorization, I told him to suggest any title he wanted, to emphasize what he thought was most important. Right here, he split the text and gave the next chapter the title...

THE PSYCHONUTRITION APPROACH

"And, if there are no fatty acids, the whole process stops?" I asked.

"It won't stop, but it is like when a machine has no oil. You know what they say: it works like a well-oiled machine. If we are not taking in enough essential fatty acids, the human body is not "lubricated" so to speak. Omegas are extremely important elements in the human diet, they are essential for our metabolic functions, and we need them every day because our bodies can't produce them themselves. Then, we also need to take the necessary quantities of minerals and vitamins. Super. We have tablets, and that is that. What else do we need? We need antioxidants. When we are losing weight, fat is broken down. Breaking it down does two things. Just by using it, it increases our metabolism. That means, on a diet, the engine is working with more revolutions, and for longer. The damage it causes is greater. The production of toxins is greater. Free radicals are created. The more we do, the more free radicals we create, so we need more antioxidants to protect our body. And we need fibre. We need to clean ourselves. We need probiotics, to maintain our intestinal flora. It would appear we have covered everything. But we haven't. The psyche! We have to find a non-food reward, something that has nothing to do with food, to reward ourselves when we achieve a result. There must be a psychological element, to stabilize our psyche. The psyche is very

Tomislav Birtić

closely related to physical chemistry. It is not possible to control hunger just like that. The question remains of appetite, the question of hunger, habits, and behaviour patterns. Here, we as professionals like to jump in with some tricks, advice, measures, to teach people, when, how much and what to eat. When we analyse the contents of a plate, it is usually a terrible mess. Messes are not resolved by fibre in tablets or a shake. It may work for a while, but sooner or later you have to go back to the beginning, the plate. We need to learn what should be on the plate, what a plate should look like. We have to learn about colours. That it is not the same if you look at a plate that is grey, over-cooked, boiled, where the colours have drained away, or if you look at something that is still green, red, attractive, and that even smells good. We should take time arranging our plate. Food demands respect. If we take a sandwich as a standard in our diet, out of laziness, we are not respecting ourselves! It matters whether our food is roast or boiled, seasoned or not. There are hot spices, and spices that warm or cool, there are exotic aromas, and they all have a function. Aromatherapy! One breath of cedar or pine can help control or reduce our appetite for food. If we arm people with this knowledge, that they sometimes do not have to eat an entire meal, that they do not need sugar after every meal, to get involved in physical activities, that at least one meal a day should be slow food, chewing slowly, and to spend an hour or an hour and a half over that meal, if they are balanced in that way, then this is an arsenal of weapons which must balance them and bring them to where they want to be. Not to go on eating after we receive the command: "Enough. I am full". We should learn something about the brain from physiology. Taken physiologically, separately and in relation to other organs, it is the organ, which, whenever it can, eats practically only sugar, it uses oxygen and behaves very selfishly, egotistically. Sometimes it is like a metabolic, monstrous, unstoppable machine, driven by sugar. After we have had something to eat, the sugar from the meal first of all goes to meet its needs, and what is left goes to the other organs. The brain uses it up very quickly and intensively, and immediately demands more. The heart, the muscles? What does it care, they can get their own supplies of energy, they can fend for themselves. It is important to understand the mechanism of sugar consumption in the body, and the cycles by which its concentration falls or rises, and who the biggest consumer of sugar in the body is. In that sense we need to understand an important lesson on winning non-food rewards. They may be an important part of the strategy of stabilizing the natural balance of blood sugar, normalizing the cycle of insulin production..."

And, Dolibašić pointed out something else in particular.

HUNGRY? SO WHAT?!

"One of the important things is to explain to people that hunger is nothing terrible. At one time people worked in the fields all day. I am hungry. So what? I will eat in an hour. Today? I am hungry. I must eat right now. A croissant and coffee. Half an hour later, let's have the same again. The modern way of life is like a mine field, and one of the mines is coffee, which today involves a fix of sugar and coffee. Insulin acts more quickly and strongly when coffee enters the scene. The euphoria that coffee creates in the body, if it is accompanied by sugar, is even stronger. The stronger the fix of sugar, the higher the peak, the climax of blood sugar concentration, the deeper the fall into hypoglycaemia. Bang, right down into hypoglycaemia. Because that insulin, when its power brings down the sugar, does not bring it down to normal levels, but below. Your hands shake. There is a nice story in the film "The Enemy of the State" with Gene Hackman and Will Smith. The former always needs sugar, he gets uptight, yells at people. When his sugar levels fall he becomes a bad man. I have actually seen people like that. If they don't get their fix of sugar, they go crazy."

As we parted, he gave me his pedometer, a step counter. And a flier, which, roughly speaking, said it all in a single sentence. "The recommended reduction in food intake is about 200-300 kcal a day, with the equivalent increase in physical activity."

BLANKA PERŠE. METABOLIC BALANCE. NOT OPRAH, NOR DR. OZ... BLANKA PERŠE

My search for the holy grail of nutrition ended with metabolic balance and Blanka Perše in the summer of 2012. After that, weighing 260-262 pounds (118-119 kilos) – for years I could not get below 253 (115), but fortunately also not above 264 (120) – it seemed as though I had never had a problem with my weight, losing 4 to 6 pounds (2 to 3 kilos) a month, going down to a little over 202 pounds (92 kilos), and then for months and months to weigh between 202 and 207 (92 and 94 kilos). From the perspective of a fatty, thinking about whether I would ever reach my ideal weight, according to the books, of 194 pounds (88 kilos), I have to remember I am over 40 years old, and 202-211 (92-96 kilos) is completely fine.

So, first the thing I am sure you want to know. Following Blanka's advice – she created a menu just for me, meaning not just that it is not for everyone, but that it is only and solely for me – I ate three meals a day. I had breakfast, lunch and evening meal – proteins with greens, plus fruit, and I had an obligatory apple every day. The last mouthful of food I ate was before nine in the evening, and as dietary supplements I took multivitamins (I already had those – a Herbalife shake, I ate or drank one, whatever, after breakfast and evening meal, or after breakfast and lunch), omega 3 (that is also in Herbalife), digestive enzymes and probiotics, which were new to my diet.

There are no words to describe the ease with which the pounds came off, and she just smiled.

As Blanka tells me, metabolic balance is a nutrition programme which does not just promote the loss of weight, but also helps with hormonal balance, by a significant increase in energy, and brings the organism to an optimal state of health. This is the result of twenty-five years of scientific work by doctors and nutritionists. Metabolic balance was never just one more diet for losing weight, but it is a life style by which slowly but surely we return to a healthy way of living. We only need to follow certain dietary rules, that is, to combine different food groups, we need good timing and a lot of good will.

To start this chapter, just an explanation of why Blanka is mentioned in the title. I am not looking for advice, nor would I give it, but I feel free to prompt people to think about the experts who are perhaps all around us, but we don't understand how important they could be. How many times, not thinking for more than a couple of seconds, we reject someone's opinion just because they are close to us? Simply because they are accessible, every day. In the end, Blanka told me about the method that was made famous by Novak Đoković about two years before the article was published in Jutarnji list and the magnificent book "Serve to Win" came out. In this book, in my humble opinion, Đoković made a greater contribution to society – mankind! – than Mohammed Ali by his activism... Of course this is nothing against Oprah, or my favourite Dr. Oz, I just want to say that knowledge is not necessarily on television, that you can find it on park benches, in lines at supermarket check outs, and knowledge about food can even be found at a dinner party where you eat too much and break all known nutrition rules...

"AFTER I GOT RID OF SUGAR FROM MY DIET MY LIFE CHANGED FOR THE BETTER"

I met Blanka Perše at a dinner party for about forty people. If such a thing as fate exists, fate would have it that we were sitting next to each other, and after a couple of topics of conversation, I told her I was writing a book about losing weight, and that I had tried out various diets on myself... And then things took off. A couple of days later I interviewed her for the book.

"From 28th December to 2nd January I gained 7 pounds (3.5 kilos). I ate after seven p.m. and I ate cakes, that is cakes as defined by the region I come from, where a cake is not a cake if it doesn't have a two pounds (kilo) of walnuts in it. I started to exercise more intensively, and in two days, since it was mainly water, I lost 4 pounds (2 kilos). What does science say, what are those 7 pounds someone puts on by eating more cakes than usual, especially after seven p.m.?" I asked.

"You said it yourself, mostly water, of course along with everything else that goes into a cake."

"What does that water bind itself to?"

"Water collects because of the toxins we bring into our organism. If we take more than usual, our bodies are not used to that quantity of toxins and can't get rid of them so easily, so the excess, bound with water, remains in our bodies. Of course, if we don't continue to eat like that, under the condition that the body is healthy, then the liquid will be slowly excreted. By all accounts, your mechanism for getting rid of toxins is pretty good. You say you exercised more intensively. So you speeded up the process. When we say "toxins" we mean food which is not good for us and which harms our organism, what may manifest itself in various ways. This problem can't be solved quickly, and people who live like that all the time have increasing health problems, such as bloatedness, water retention in various parts of their bodies, problems with their kidneys, liver and heart... It lasts for years, but people often think they have fallen ill overnight. No one gets ill overnight."

"What would be a typical example of getting ill over many years?"

"Let's say, sugar consumption. By eating sugar people don't just get diabetes. Sugar is bad, bad, bad. In our house we don't even have a sugar bowl, I don't use it at all. When I was young, when I didn't know what I know now, I ate a lot of sugar. We ate cakes every day. And my health suffered as a result. I didn't get a single disease we can name. I didn't get diabetes, nor even any disturbance of the glucose in my blood, or blood sugar as people like to call it, but I had a thousand other problems. I got headaches, I was tired, I even had periods of mild depression. Until I got rid of sugar from my diet, I didn't feel any improvement. I stopped using sugar in my diet for the first time when I was studying nutrition in 1994. And I noticed a change. Still, I very quickly returned to my sugar using habit. Because we quickly become extremely dependent on sugar, it is like a drug, but today we know that sugar is poison. In the end, after I stopped eating sugar, my life changed for the better. What can you get from sugar? The results, to mention just a few, may be excess weight, diabetes,

Tomislav Birtić

dementia (today we call it diabetes 3), heart disease, kidney problems, hormonal disorders, various forms of carcinomas..."

"SOMETIME YOU PUT ON WEIGHT SIMPLY BECAUSE YOU ARE RETAINING WATER, BUT YOU RETAIN IT FOR A THOUSAND REASONS"

"I hiked nineteen miles (thirty-two kilometres). A climb of about 700 metres, and the same again down-hill, all together eight and a half hours at a temperature of 96 Fahrenheit (36 degrees). I expected that I would lose weight from all that physical effort, that I would lose pounds. But I became bloated, I put 6. I asked the doctor what had happened to me. He told me that I had retained water in my body. But how could I retain water when I sweated so much?" I asked Blanka.

"It is hard to say off the top of my head. However similar we all are, our health is determined by our biochemical diversity. I don't know your organism. I can only guess. Perhaps there is an imbalance in your hormonal system, which is very important for regulating water in your body. Also the kidneys are involved in the process, since, along with the liver, they remove toxins from your body. There may be some imbalance in your digestive system, which I think is the most important factor in your diet. The imbalance may mean that there are more bad bacteria in your intestines than good, it may mean having parasites rather than not having any or having very few, imbalance may mean having a yeast infection, and so on. A bad diet causes an increase in all these negative factors. The body will then not function well, and it will do the opposite of what it should do."

Tomislav Birtić

"Was the water retention helped by the fact that it was the first major effort of that kind I had subjected my body to, since it was used to climbing for just two or three hours?"

"It was definitely stressful for your body. If we are under stress, the adrenal gland works faster, producing adrenalin. What does adrenalin do? Amongst other things, adrenalin gives us strength to walk those nineteen miles. In order to have the strength, we need glucose, the only form of sugar that functions as food for our brain and all our cells. And it will be released when there are reserves to supply the organism. That process may lead to an imbalance in the entire hormonal system, including the pituitary gland, which is involved in regulating water in the body. And the prime mover of it all is stress."

"Did I get my body into such a state that it was defending itself from me? Did my unhappy organism think: 'This idiot is trying to kill me, now I have to protect all the reserves I have to survive', and defend itself from me?"

"That's right. Hormones are important in regulating water. The kidneys and all that is related to the digestive system. However, in a stressful situation the digestive system shuts down, so we don't use energy on digesting food. And as far as the sporting element is concerned... You probably know that a certain percentage of sportsmen get sick. People wonder why. How can such a great sportsman, so strong and healthy, get, for instance, cancer? Due to the increased levels of stress he was subject to during training."

"Man, you mean, he may think he is enjoying sport, but actually the spirit of the man thinks an activity is pleasant, but the body of the man is actually suffering?"

"Precisely! The man is enjoying himself, but his body is under stress. His organism is under stress. And, now, if that goes on for a long time... Imagine how many years and how many hours sportsmen and women train every day. This does not mean in any way that training means you will get sick, but if they don't eat well, their bodies have a hard time dealing with all that stress. That is why they need help to deal with the stress. Antioxidants play an important role in that: vitamins A, C and E, and selenium, magnesium and B vitamins."

"My father started smoking when he was forty, and he smoked until he was in his sixties. He was in very poor condition. First of all he started walking. After walking was no effort for him anymore, he started to jog, at first running steps half the length of his foot. And so, by doing something that was not any effort for him, he trained himself to lift hundred and ten pounds (fifty kilos) with no strain, to run six miles (ten kilometres), and if the lift wasn't working he would climb up to the fifteenth floor carrying a weight like it was nothing... Perhaps the definition of recreation is only activities which are pleasant for your body, whilst sport is any activity that raises your pulse, let's say, above one hundred and forty."

"I would agree with that. We tell people that they should exercise at least three times a week for twenty minutes: fast walking or running. Recreation is really fun, but in sport you want to achieve something."

"When I started exercising, I couldn't even walk a mile without a break. My physiotherapist said that then even normal walking was like training for me, because when I walked my pulse would go up to 120-

Tomislav Birtić

130. Her definition of training is actually the pulse rate."

"Pulse rate is extremely important in exercise, that's true."

"What do you think of L-Carnitine?"

"All amino acids, the smallest protein molecules we can absorb, are very important for our organism. Just as glucose gives energy, proteins are like building bricks for our body. And L-Carnitine, like other amino acids, is important for energy, because energy can't be produced if, amongst other things there is not enough L-Carnitine. It is good for sportsmen and women, and for people who have problems with their heart, because they do not produce enough energy."

"It helped me a lot for three weeks. The doctors and physiotherapists told me I shouldn't take it for more than three weeks at a time, and they told me the longer I exercise, the better it works. Instead of an hour, I would walk quickly for two hours, and I melted away. Just with Nordic walking. OK – four to five miles (seven to eight) kilometres an hour. Two hours' Nordic walking a day and I melted away so much it was visible in the mirror. However, two months later, after the recommended break, L-Carnitine no longer worked on me at all. Why?"

"I believe in the ability of the organism to reject some things if it doesn't need them. Probably you didn't need it any more, or it would have done you harm if you had taken it. You can take as much vitamin C as you like, your body will use as much as it needs, and will reject the excess."

"STRESS IS NUMBER ONE IN OUR LIVES. IF PEOPLE WOULD ACCEPT THAT, AS WELL AS EATING HEALTHILY, EVERY ONE WOULD MEDITATE"

"One more mystery. Why does sleeping help us lose weight? If I managed to fall asleep at ten or eleven at night, my weight loss would be visible, but when I couldn't sleep, or even if I just went to bed late without insomnia, either I didn't lose weight or I lost weigh much more slowly..."

"Stress. Stress. In my opinion, stress is number one in our lives. If people knew that, as well as eating healthily, everyone would meditate."

"What is worst, no one has defined it."

"I can tell you what happens in a physiological sense. Stress is a natural mechanism, vital and useful. I don't know if you have heard of the "fight or flight" syndrome. It is an automatic, primitive physiological reaction, which prepares our body to fight or fly, in a situation where our life is in danger. The hypothalamus sends a message to the adrenalin glands to produce adrenalin and cortisol, which then send a message to the entire organism to get ready either to fight or fly. Our pupils widen, so we can see better, our digestive system closes down, because we shouldn't waste our energy, our heart and breathing speed up. In stressful situations people are capable of doing incredible things..."

"Yes, mothers lift trucks..."

Tomislav Birtić

"Of course there is also a psychological element. If a mother sees her child under a truck, her strength increases incredibly, which is also an example of the fight syndrome. But, what was actually happening? Prepared for new situations, we fought or we escaped and used up the energy, and returned to a balance state of rest. We did everything our body was prepared for. What happens today? Your boss annoys you at work, there is a tram hold up and you are late, you can't either fight or fly, so you get tense and aggressive, and you are ready to explode at any moment. You have not used up that energy, got rid of it."

"So, the energy package was ready, it was not used up, so it was just stored?"

"Precisely! Day after day. That is how we live. What happens then? From acute stress we move on to chronic stress. We can no longer see a way out of the desperate situation. The worst aspect of chronic stress is that people get used to it and are no longer aware of it. You probably know the story about how during a war, when they were all subject to chronic stress, people mainly do not get ill. The stress keeps them in a state of tension all the time. And, not only do they not get ill, but the chronic illnesses they have suddenly become milder. Why?"

"Their coordinate system has shifted?"

"That's right. After the war, when their hormone levels fall, people start getting terribly ill, because their bodies are exhausted from the long-term stress."

"Like journalists on holiday."

"That's right. Chronic stress destroys people's lives, in an unhappy marriage, at a job they don't like, in a difficult life. People, who have done a stressful job all their lives, think that when they retire they will relax and rest, but actually they often suffer a heart attack or get ill. Because the mechanism of stress is no longer protecting them, or they are completely exhausted."

"From all you are saying, it seems that we should start meditating at the latest from our sixteenth birthday, or at least see a good psychologist."

"TM or any other form of meditation has a cumulative effect. At first you feel great while you are meditating, but as time passes, meditation becomes an increasing part of your life. You feel good all day."

"That means, you recommend either psychology, or meditation, or let's say, any form of technique to clear your mind?"

"Precisely. Or rest. It is important to teach our brain that it can rest, that it doesn't need to work all the time. We should "feed" our bodies with meditation every day, like food."

And then Blanka told me everything I wanted to know about food supplements, in a couple of sentences. Actually, if necessary, it would all fit into one sentence.

"THE MINIMUM OF MINIMUMS OF FOOD SUPPLEMENTS FOR OUR TIME: VITAMIN C, OMEGA 3, MULTIVITAMINS, DIGESTIVE ENZYMES AND PROBIOTICS"

"What does a nutritionist have to say about food supplements?"

"There are many different opinions."

"How can I help someone? How can someone know what he should take and what he shouldn't? You see, we have an uneducated person, who sees an advertisement with a fat guy on one side and the ideal of beauty on the other, and in the corner a box of something with a Latin name. How can a layperson find his way around that nightmare?"

"Lay people know nothing about that. That is why there are nutritionists. People watch advertisements, they read things, and they get completely lost. With pollution as it is today, food is no longer healthy like it used to be. You can't take food supplements just like that, because some may be bad for your health if they are not under control, but everyone should take some vitamin C, omega 3, a good multivitamin with a high percentage of vitamin B, digestive enzymes and probiotics. This is the minimum of minimums, which everyone needs to maintain their health. We don't get enough omega 3 in our diet, and its most important effect is anti-inflammatory. As every imbalance in the organism leads to an inflammation to a greater or lesser degree, omega 3 is vital. From multivitamins our body takes what it needs, and we should take digestive enzymes so our pancreas is not overstrained by our digestive system, because it has enough work to do with insulin. Some people are afraid that our body will become lazy if we take them and stop producing its own enzymes. It won't get lazy. In fact, we will help it to use energy on something that is more important at any given moment. Today we also know that enzymes enter the blood and clean it from everything that is not good. The more of them there are, the more they will clean. But the story doesn't end there. There are two main groups of enzymes: digestive and metabolic. Digestive enzymes, which we can take orally, ease the burden on the metabolic enzymes, and metabolic enzymes are the decisive factor in many processes that take place in our bodies. So, when we take digestive enzymes, we are literally extending our life."

"But how much should we take?"

"They won't do you any harm. I always have them with me. When we start to eat a meal, we take some digestive enzyme, and then it is only for our digestion. Between meals they are taken as therapy, depending on the diagnosis."

Tomislav Birtić

"CONSULT A NUTRITIONIST, BECAUSE YOU ARE NOT WHAT YOU EAT, BUT WHAT YOU ABSORB"

"A lot of advertisements say 'consult your doctor', 'before you go on a diet, go and see your doctor'... Most people say that they know everything they need to know about losing weight, and it comes down to 'eat less and exercise'. However, my research showed what you suffer if you think you can do it by yourself. What do you, as a nutritionist, have to say about the most common mistakes people make because they don't seek the advice of an expert?"

"There are so many.... Let us go back to the fact that we are all different. They say that before you go on a diet you should go to a doctor for a check-up, and I would add that you should also go to a nutritionist. You don't know what problems you have. Good digestion is a must for good health, because food has to pass through your digestive tract. I can't even begin to list all the problems you could have here. They say that you are what you eat, but what is actually true is that you are what you absorb. You can eat the best food in the world, but if your digestive tract is not able to digest it, and then absorb it... There is something known as "leaky gut". Because you eat badly, the walls of your intestines become too porous, and food that should not get in to our organism, gets absorbed. Chaos occurs in our body, because we don't know what to do with those huge molecules that don't belong there. Therefore our immune system begins to attack them, and that is precisely one of the factors that cause autoimmune diseases. Of course we have to check up on the condition of the heart, liver and kidneys. So, you have to go to see a doctor and a nutritionist, because there may be many problems in your body, that you don't know about if there are no symptoms."

"My friend brought me Montignac, and told me that the entire book is contained in two pages. They contain a graph showing why we get hungry quickly, and a page telling us which food should be combined with which other food. The rest of the book, my friend joked, was written because he couldn't just sell those two pages, he had to write at least a hundred. So I concluded that often I didn't put on weight because of food, meals, but because of snacks. When I started to be careful about snacks, when those snacks became either almonds or a Herbalife protein bar, or a shake, with some light exercise, let's say three to four miles (five to seven kilometres) a day, I lost 11 pounds (5 kilos) a week, and I wasn't hungry. Not even 'I eat, so I lose weight', but 'I snack, so I lose weight', and I even had phases when 'I gorge myself, and lose weight', because I was careful what I combined with what, and I was exercising a lot. For instance, for supper: tuna with Swiss chard in unlimited quantities."

"You ate as much as you wanted?"

"Yes, I ate as much as I wanted, but I didn't put on weight, I lost weight. Is it a case of my individual organism, for which this was coincidently suitable, or does this story indicate a universal truth?"

"I am always for the individual approach. Some people have to eat snacks to maintain normal sugar levels in their blood."

Tomislav Birtić

"Did I provide my body with sufficient glucose by snacking, that is, eating healthy snacks, unconsciously, without any idea of what I was doing? And my body said, gratefully, 'Thank goodness, he remembered'?"

"I wouldn't put it like that, it would be better to say you gave your body an even quantity of glucose. In that way, you maintain your energy, that is, your body produces enough energy for the entire day."

"You mean to say, I enable it to get rid of its excess in peace? To say: 'I don't need to panic, to pack things away, I can get rid of these excesses'."

"Your body says: 'See how well I am doing, now I have a continuous supply of fuel for sufficient energy'. People drink a lot of coffee. Why? Because they need energy. After every cup of coffee, their adrenalin glands raise their energy levels by producing adrenalin for a short period of time. The suddenness of the burst of energy also means it quickly falls."

"You mean, like a drug fix? Like strong liquor? Are we talking about sugar as a drug again?"

"Precisely. And when it suddenly falls again, people become aggressive, irritable and hungry, so they need more sugar in the form of a stimulant, like coffee, alcohol, a carbonized drink, or food rich in carbohydrates, such as bread, pasta or cakes. And then the problem of insulin is linked with this, as in this situation it raises the inflammation in the organism. When sugar levels rise suddenly, each time you get, as you say a fix, insulin knocks at the door of the cells to let glucose into every cell in our body. The cell only takes as much glucose as it needs, whilst it converts the rest into fat and that is stored in the body."

"So this would be how it goes.... I am a journalist. I have been under incredible stress for months. I come to work, and I am immediately hungry. I eat, let's say, eggs and ham. My snacks are always sandwiches. My brain is occupied all the time, and my body is screaming, 'Give me sugar, rescue me!' And it all gets stored round my waist."

"Precisely. The next step is insulin resistance. Imagine that you are continuously overloading an engine. It will work for a while, and then it will start to go wrong and finally stop. That is how it is with insulin. Due to frequent use and overload it can no longer be as efficient as before, and more and more needs to be produced for the same effect. In the worst case scenario it leads to diabetes, malignant disease, and a whole range of serious chronic illnesses."

Before we get onto kinesiology or human kinetics, that Blanka told me about two years before Đoković made gluten free food and kinesiology famous, one more thing.

"ACIDITY= ILLNESS, ALKALINITY= ILLNESS. WE WERE CREATED FOR A BALANCE BETWEEN ALKALINITY AND ACIDITY"

"Why do protein and starch, let's say, meat and chips, have a horrible result, but meat and Swiss chard have a good result?"

"Because Swiss chard is alkaline and meat is acidic. That is, I think, one of the most important aspects of diet. If we eat acid food, it does not mean that the food has an acid taste, but that the food creates acid in our body, we are talking about the pH factor. Acidity increases and acidity is the same as illness. If we eat alkaline food, if we reduce the acidity, then we bring the pH factor back towards normal. It is always better to be a little more alkaline than acidic. If we eat potatoes and meat, which both create acid in the organism, that is not good, because acidity has a cumulative effect and therefore increases the degree of illness. We should always eat vegetables. Vegetables are fantastic. They say we should eat five meals of vegetables and fruit a day. I would say, five meals of vegetables a day! We can eat the best piece of meat, and it still creates a high level of acidity, because its pH factor is between 1.5 and 2. But if we eat a heap of vegetables and salad with that meat, we will balance the acidity.

"My friends come over, to watch a match. For years it has been the same, crisps and beer. Now I get them crisps and beer, as the host, but during the match I eat broccoli. They think it is hilarious. But I eat broccoli from my mum's garden."

"Fantastic!"

"OK, I do drink a bit of beer, but I have cut it down incredibly. If I don't eat broccoli, while they are eating crisps, I eat almonds, because I have realized that if I eat about one hundred grams of almonds in the evening, they do weigh a bit heavy on my stomach, but it is not a big deal. Proteins help expel water, but almonds don't get stuck on my waist, they don't create new pounds."

"And they are alkaline."

"That means, one hundred grams of almonds are six hundred calories. Let's say I ate one thousand two hundred calories of chocolate, it will be seen immediately as a 3 pounds (kilo and a half) excess weight, because over a night or two some processes have to take place in the body that result in putting on weight, whilst one thousand two hundred calories of almonds may even mean losing a 2 pounds (kilo)."

"Because they contain proteins. The digestive system always takes longer if you eat proteins, although it would not be good to eat so many almonds. Your body needs four hours to digest proteins. Carbohydrates wait for the proteins. That is why you should eat proteins with every meal. If we eat an apple, it is good to eat four or five almonds with it."

"To feel full for two to three hours?"

"To feel full, and to allow glucose to enter your blood slowly."

"Why is breakfast so important? Why, if you haven't eaten anything, should you at least drink a glass of water?"

"Again, this is our old friend, stress. You were sleeping, everything was peaceful. As soon as you get up, your body is immediately 'wound up'. As long as you don't eat any food, it is producing adrenalin, which releases glucose from the organism, to have energy, because we are active."

"Does our entire life really come down to providing glucose?"

"Yes. It is the only thing that gives us energy. However, we now know new things in relation to producing energy, but that is a whole new chapter."

"If someone doesn't have breakfast, where does his organism get its energy?"

"From his muscles, in the form of glycogen."

"Why doesn't it take it from fat?"

"When the reserves of glycogen are used up, the body turns to its fat reserves. Fat is a reserve for bad times."

"I HAD ABSOLUTELY NO CONTROL OVER MY ARM AND I WAS AMAZED EVERY TIME IT REMAINED LOCKED"

Now all I have left to do is write about what kinesiology is, that is, what Blanka told me about two years before Đoković published his book "Serve to Win". Unfortunately on the day when Blanka, who lives in London, was in Zagreb and had time to do a kinesiology examination of my sister and me, I had some unavoidable commitments. So she only examined Marija, who told me all about it...

"After I lay down on my back on the massage table, Blanka tested my supraspinatus, a muscle in my right arm, by pushing my arm in a certain direction, and I had to resist. Since the muscle was unbalanced, she had no problem moving my arm despite my resistance. The next step was to test certain substances to find the one that is important for balancing this muscle. She put one product group after another on my neck, to see what was lacking in my organism. She started with products for immunity. After the product had been placed on my neck, I would stretch out my right arm, with a firm and straight elbow, and when Blanka said 'resistance' I would push my arm away from my body and she would push it towards me. If my arm was firm, Blanka could not move it even by pushing hard, which meant that I needed that product. It is a completely uncontrolled, involuntary, unconscious reaction of the organism. I had absolutely no control over my arm, although

Tomislav Birtić

I tried, and I was amazed every time when my arm locked and was incredibly firm, although it is mine, part of my body. Just as in integrative psychology, or core energetics, I was surprised, thinking that I knew my body better, but actually I have no idea about my body, or about my internal, unconscious world. She told me that when someone comes for their first examination, she takes a medical history and talks with the patient about why they came, or about their health problems. The first examination is more about what the organism needs physically, from a nutrition point of view. Later, after the organism has become stronger, by taking different substances – the things it is lacking, systematic kinesiology therapy also includes reprogramming internal psycho-emotional patterns. She told me about that, but she hasn't done that with me yet. She worked on neurovascular and lymphatic systems, and meridians, using ancient Chinese medicine techniques. It was quite painful, because a lot of "rubbish" had accumulated in those points, toxins, due to my poor diet, negative emotions, or structural problems. Regular therapy also includes expelling various toxins from the body. The body has a lot of points, through which individual organs can be treated, as well as the toxins built up in our organs and the areas surrounding them. To put it simply, the entire body is bound together as a system, and is as healthy as the least healthy part. A systematic examination can establish precisely where the organism is 'weakest', that is what is the priority in the body, and of all its problems, what needs to be focused on first (urgently). If for example I was physically healthy, and Blanka told me that she had a client who was physically super, and didn't need anything, then we could move to the next level. But that is rare, most people have some weaknesses in terms of nutrition.

After that she tested a few other muscles, mainly related to immunity, which was my main problem, and the appropriate treatment. At the end of the session, the conclusion was that my organism needed vitamin C, two products to strengthen my immunity, digestive enzymes and several types of Bach drops. After I had taken these products for a while, since the examination had shown that they were the priority for me, the overall condition of my organism improved. I felt better in myself, I had more energy.

Before the examination and taking those products, my nails were really fragile. I remember I was frightened because if I held something tight, white lines would appear on my nails, as though they had split width ways. I also had a lot of hangnails, and the skin around my nails would peal. By taking those products, this all cleared up, and I felt more stable, both physically and emotionally."

Tomislav Birtić

DEALING WITH MY EMOTIONS HELPED
ME LOSE WEIGHT

I contemplated about what to have for breakfast before going for a swim.

"None of that does any good until you deal with the emotions that make you gain weight," my sister Marija mentioned in passing. She couldn't stand watching me any more choosing what I was not going to have for breakfast. Yes... People usually choose what they will have for breakfast. But those of use who suffer with our weight, and struggle with ourselves, we choose what we are not going to eat.

At the seaside I didn't feel like cooking, I rationalized that I had had enough salad, and mozzarella, and my brother-in-law makes the best sandwiches on the face of the earth, the best barbecue, and then we went out for dinner that evening, a little risotto... Add a beer or two, a bit of pasta, you can swim as much as you like, but there I was again, weighing 260 pounds (118 kilos).

Marija is nine years younger than me. And, when you take the fact that immediately after she had started studying integrative psychology, she was already the smartest person on earth – and you combine that with the age difference, it is very true that for about twenty years I did try not to react in the heat of the moment, but in the end you get something like a boiling pot. And then she added...

"You see, you don't understand it now. You can't understand it, so we won't talk about it now. But when you realize that you can be a thousand times disciplined and lose weight with a huge effort, but you will still put the weight back on again, unless you work on the emotions which always make you fall and give up, because you can't hold everything inside like you are, so you fill the hole with food, you compensate with food, you come and tell me when you have understood what it is all about. And now have whatever you like for breakfast, and go have a swim. While you are swimming, try to do something useful. Think about what makes you gorge yourself on ten toasted sandwiches after ten at night, after you have made such an effort to lose weight. That will help you more than guarano."

I opened my mouth. I wanted to argue, but Marija didn't want to know. She simply cut me off, saying I could not understand it now, that it was impossible for me to understand at that time, because emotions are more powerful than reason, and in those circumstances there is no sense in wasting time. In her school they learnt that people like me can rationalize everything to death, but, she repeated, there was no point, and that she bet anything I liked that I would come to her soon, because I would definitely understand and apply the principles they learnt in school.

Perhaps I was still hot on holiday. Even while I was swimming that the first time, after the hint she gave me, right up to the end of the holiday, I still didn't get it. I didn't understand the connection between emotions and what I was doing. My mind was enough.

But when I was hiking in the mountains, alone with myself and the beautiful fragrances of nature, I thought about the things that worried me most. Above all my other worries, I singled out my concern that I could possibly lose part or most of my income.

Tomislav Birtić

Since I had survived three years of starvation, horrible starvation, getting even slightly close to that concept upset me horribly.

Not to go into details, the method that Marija used to help me with to deal with my emotions, not the loss of part or most of my income, nor the extinction of an entire branch... After I had dealt with my fear of losing my living, alcohol disappeared from my life, as though it had never been there. Make no mistake, I am not a drunkard, but I would have a couple of drinks with my friends, almost every day. That damn sugar alcohol, that cursed rise in insulin levels and its consequences. In some episodes of losing weight, I would succeed in abstaining, yes, I resisted when I was in a café. But then I would suddenly put back on the pounds I had lost. And then, literally unconsciously, I went into a café and ordered a coffee and water. And then I went again and again to different cafés, and ordered coffee and water. Deal with emotions – thank you, sister! – this meant that I no longer had the need for two drinks a day, and in many situations I found alcohol repulsive. I would only drink a glass of wine in the best company, and I truly enjoyed it. Alcohol no longer mastered me, but I actually controlled my fear, and I mastered the alcohol.

Truth, the whole truth and nothing but the truth. In company we would drink eight rounds. Somewhere around the seventh they would ask me how I could drink so much coffee and mineral water. I would reply that they were actually right, and just when their faces were getting red, when they thought they I would finally order something stronger, I told them that I would forget the coffee, and that plain water is better than fizzy.

I THINK THE BEST BOOKS ON LOSING WEIGHT ARE ACTUALLY NOT BOOKS ON LOSING WEIGHT

This book is like an unplanned, conceived child, whose conception the parents, who love each other, welcome with excitement, enthusiasm, and you can see from miles away that the child will always be loved, adored. And it is. There is no but.

Indeed, I did not plan to write a book about losing weight. It never entered my mind that I would ever write a book about losing weight. The idea occurred to me when I had slimmed down from 295 (134) to 229 pounds (104 kilos). I told my friends jokingly that, after biographies, sagas, novels and manifestos, I would finally write something that was useful for people. My friends fell about laughing. One of the objections was how would anyone believe my novel, after a book on losing weight. I said that there is no question about believing or not believing in a cure for a disease. It either cures the disease or it doesn't. And it does not matter if the cure was written by the author of a book on losing weight, or a doctor or pharmacologist with fifty years of experience in his field, who took good care not to ruin his reputation by writing an unsuitable booklet.

Just as it did not occur to me in my wildest dreams that I would ever write a book about losing weight, it also never occurred to me that the book would take almost eight years to complete. I put on weight, I weighed 295 pounds (134 kilos), and suddenly and without expert advice (unhealthily!) I went down to 229 (104). Euphoric, optimistic, I did not believe I would put that weight on again, that I would struggle for years between 253 (115) and 264 pounds (120 kilos), or that my search for a map leading me to victory would take so long. And that is what this entire chapter is about. I mean that the child, like any child, went out of control, and after all those years I have to say that this is not a book about losing weight. What I actually want to say is...

One of those people who take up two seats in a plane was standing by the shelves with the top 100 non-fiction books in the bookshop at Gatwick airport. I don't know if the 100 best-selling books were displayed on the shelf or 100 recommendations. But the first and second in the list of non-fiction were books on losing weight.

And so at first he was just looking, looking and looking at those two books, but he did not pick them up. Then he took the first one off the shelf. He looked at the cover, flicked through it, and put it back. He took the second one, and went through the same procedure. He walked a few feet away, looked at the non-fiction and the fiction, and then went back to the books on losing weight. This time he studied them thoroughly. Foreword, post-word, randomly opened any page and read it. To cut a long story short, he walked around the shop for about twenty minutes, looked at bags, then the books, T-shirts, then the books, and in the end he bought both of them...

Ha! Even before I read Ðoković's book "Serve to Win", with the subtitle "The 14-Day Gluten-Free Plan for Physical and Mental Excellence", I told my friends that the best book I had ever read on losing weight was not a book on losing weight at all, but "Mayo Clinic's Fitness for Everybody". Of course it goes without saying that I don't think that exercise without a diet will solve the problem, but you understand what I want to say. The child went out of control the moment I became able to form a sentence saying I think the best books on losing weight are actually not books on losing weight, but about a change in life habits, about choosing life instead of a form of dying or self-destruction, whatever.

I dare to say that there are two methods. The first is without movement, with strict control of calorie intake. The second method is – I can be a glutton but lose weight. OK, I am not a glutton, but after I slimmed down from 295 pounds (134) kilos to 202 (92), there were many evening meals when I ate three rich chocolate cakes. My chubby friends would look at me almost with tears in their eyes, and ask what the secret of my success was, how was it that at ten in the evening I could eat a Wiener schnitzel, salad and three pieces of chocolate cake, wash them down with two glasses of wine, and still remain slim. I would tell them the truth, the whole truth and nothing but the truth. Every month I walk at least one sixty miles (hundred kilometres), sometimes one hundred eighty (three hundred), I do press-ups and sit-ups, and whenever I can I hike in the mountains. Sometimes the terrain is very difficult, and keeping balance requires extreme effort, let alone climbing and descending, and I walk for about ten hours. True, I take breaks. And there are not many evening meals when I eat a steak, pasta, salad, three pieces of cake and drink two glasses of wine. No more than once a week.

Tomislav Birtić

The child has got out of control and wants to get out into the world. I could write a zillion other things. As you go you hear that green tea has zero calories, but your body, in order to conquer it, burns fifty calories a cup. Two cups a day, that is three thousand calories a month, as though you don't eat anything for a day and a half.

I tried gluten-free food. I didn't need two weeks, as Đoković writes, to feel a fantastic change for the better in only four days.

Yes, the book also lacks a chapter on eating raw food. I love raw food. I have some tools for that kind of food as well, for instance: a peeler for making spaghetti from courgettes, carrots or cucumbers, which you then cover with a sauce of soya milk, almonds and other things. Fantastic! Cakes made from raw food are great too.

More than calories, I take care of the nutritional needs of my body. With calories or pounds, it's easy. But for years I had no idea how important the things were that the body needs in milligrams....

Yes, the best books on losing weight are not actually books on losing weight, I thought, and realized that I had cleaned up my body so well, that a second beer was too much for me. Believe it or not, I, who was once able to drink five beers, thinking it had no effect on me, can now only drink two beers after hours and hours of hiking in the mountains, and only if the company is perfect, as it is in the mountains. But the company at dinner is sometimes such that I drink a bottle of wine on my own, but those are rare Fridays. One glass is just right.

I eat almost no bread. Only occasionally. Rolls even less. I was overjoyed to find that a third roll made me feel sick. Nauseous, I felt like I was drunk.

In the end it's all obvious. Even the story about the fact that I want to help people, but I wouldn't mind at all if by helping people I make a million dollars. But I would be happiest if I got the odd compliment saying that this is actually not a book about losing weight. That the book is great, but that it is not a book about losing weight, but about something much more.

Tomislav Birtić

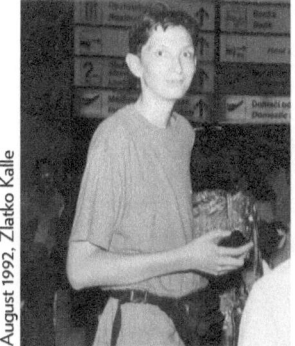

August 1992, Zlatko Kalle

Sometimes life really gets to you. This is me in the summer of 1992. I starved for a long time, not because I wanted to be thin, but because I didn't have anything to eat. I have no idea how much I weighed then.

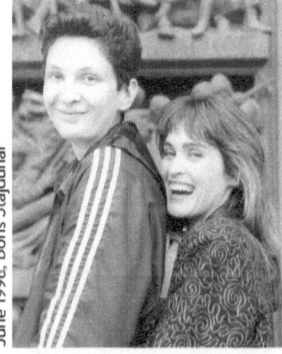

June 1996, Boris Štajduhar

Four years later, you might say, life was good to me. I am posing in Milan in the company of famous model Bernarda Marovt, and at twenty-six I looked like a school kid. My career was going well.

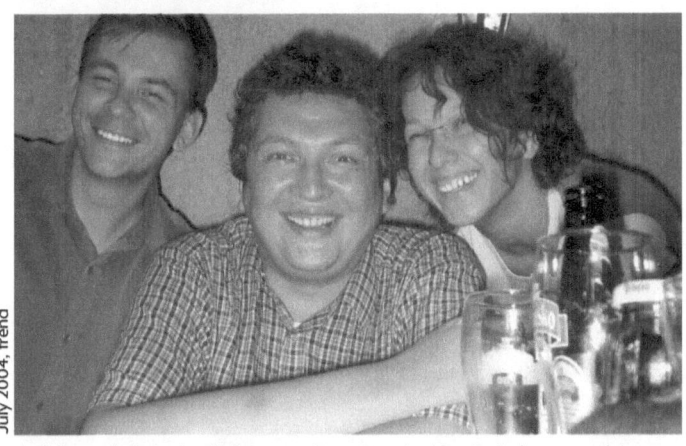

July 2004, frend

And then, a little work, a little stress, depression, bad food, a little too much hanging out in cafés... and then, it's not so bad that people no longer recognize you, but – you can't even recognize yourself.

I LOST 90 POUNDS FOR GOOD

January 2005, Stjepan Banović

July 2005, Stjepan Banović

October 2007, Stjepan Banović

January 2011, Zdeslav Barač

March 2007, Jasmin Krpan

Tomislav Birtić

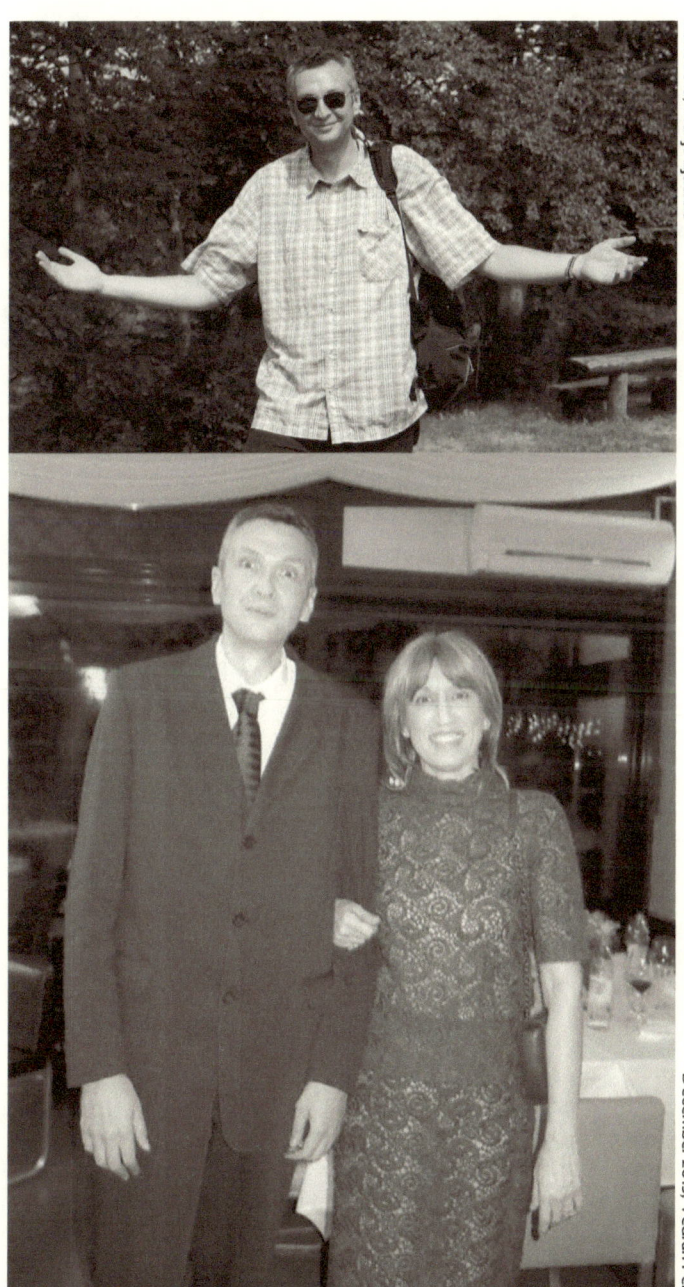

June 2013, Marija Ljubičić

December 2013, Vedran Perše

July 2013, Ivana Šoljan

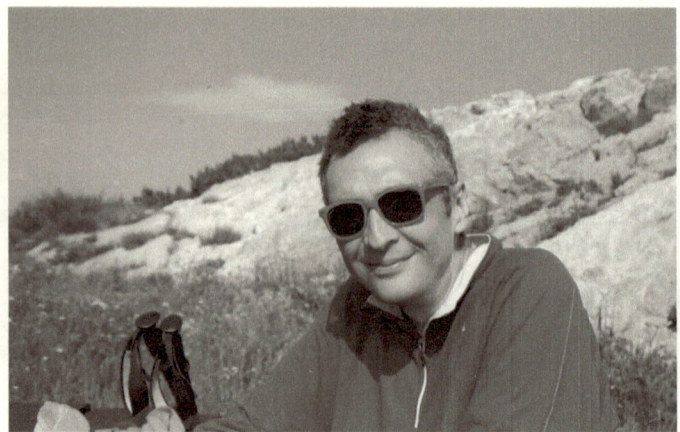

They say the answers to the same questions don't change with time. But they actually do. Here, what should be said is that I have worked for all the most important and biggest Croatian newspapers, and I have so far published nine books. However, what has changed, I mean, the most important fact about me, is that for me the most important information is the weather forecast for one mountain or another. The photograph is of the re-born me taken on Risnjak.

Tomislav Birtić

CONTENT

Tomislav Birtić
I LOST 90 POUNDS FOR GOOD

PUBLISHER
Tomislav Birtić

TRANSLATED INTO ENGLISH
Janet Tuškan

DESIGN
Gabrijela Farčić

PHOTOGRAPHS
Stjepan Banović, Zdeslav Barač, Zlatko Kalle, Jasmin Krpan,
Marija Ljubičić, Vedran Perše, Ivana Šoljan, Boris Štajduhar

ISBN-13 978-1505747522
ISBN-10 150574752X